D0921324

Changing the Game Plan
The Trey Rood Story

Trey Rood and Cherie Rood
with Donna Gentry Morton

www.prayfortrey.org

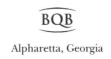

Alpharetta, Georgia

Changing the Game Plan: The Trey Rood Story
© 2014 Trey Rood and Cherie Rood. All rights reserved.

No part of this book may be reproduced in any form or by any means, electronic, mechanical, digital, photocopying, or recording, except for the inclusion in a review, without permission in writing from the publisher.

We have tried to re-create events, locales, and conversations from our memories of them.

This book is not intended as a substitute for the medical advice of physicians. The reader should regularly consult a physician in matters relating to his/her health and particularly with respect to any symptoms that may require diagnosis or medical attention.

Published in the United States by BQB Publishing
(Boutique of Quality Books Publishing Company)
www.bqbpublishing.com

Printed in the United States of America

978-1-939371-49-2 (p)
978-1-939371-50-8 (e)

Library of Congress Control Number: 2014932878

Book design by Robin Krauss, bookformatters.com.
Cover design by Dave Grauel, davidgrauel.com.
Cover photograph by Kristy Dickerson, www.kristydickerson.com.

Great appreciation goes to family friend Erik Stauber for his contribution to the cover design.

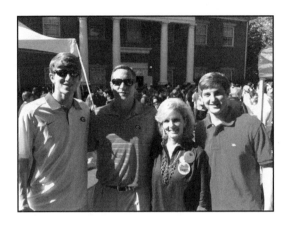

Foreword

It's often said that cancer doesn't discriminate. It can also be said that cancer doesn't isolate.

Nobody is more affected than the person who hears the words "You have cancer." But everyone who knows and loves that person feels the effects in some manner, whether they're only part of the journey for a short while, or walk the path every step. Cancer somehow changes, inspires, touches, or motivates each of these people.

There are many books written from the perspective of the patient, and many penned by a single caregiver or observer. Few, though, encompass the thoughts and feelings of a teenage cancer survivor. Even fewer are written through the eyes of several family members and friends. What they see and how they feel are their own unique and personal stories.

Cancer can reshape a life, redefine the word "normal," and challenge the very core of the person on a mission to survive. These people do not travel alone, though, and those who share their paths have voices too. Together, they all contribute to tell the story of survival.

Trey Rood and Cherie Rood
March 2014
www.prayfortrey.org

PART I

Chapter One

Trey Rood

No child should have to think about cancer, even at fifteen. They do think about it, though, because they hear a lot about it. A friend's parent is diagnosed, a teacher gets the bad news, or a neighbor down the street goes into treatment. Sometimes it strikes closer to home and someone in their own family is told they have it.

So, while fifteen-year-olds do think about life-threatening diseases, it's usually because they see it happening to someone else. They don't think about having one themselves, and never expect to be the one to hear "You have cancer."

My name is Trey Rood, and I turned fifteen in February 2007. In the days just before my birthday, I was thinking about baseball a lot. I had just made the junior varsity team at South Forsyth High School in Cumming, Georgia, which is about twenty-five miles northeast of Atlanta.

As a freshman, making junior varsity was a big deal to me, giving me a chance to play up, to challenge my game. During my entire freshman year of high school, I went to some kind of athletic practice straight after school, and there was not a single day when I was the first to leave. In the fall, I played football; in the winter, I played basketball. Come that spring, I would be playing junior varsity baseball.

As a young athlete, though, football was my favorite sport and the one I hoped to play throughout high school, maybe into college.

I was feeling pretty good about everything in life. The only thing that seemed out of place was a small lump behind my right ear. It was about the size of a regular marble, on the same side where I'd had a mole removed from the right side of my face when I was nine years old. Still, it wasn't anything I was stressing over. Back then, my family dermatologist, Dr. Michael Fisher of Atlanta Center for Dermatologic Disease, originally took a biopsy of my suspicious mole, then sent me to a plastic surgeon. My family and I didn't think much about the fact that pathology doctors consulted three times before agreeing the mole had a clear baseline. The pathology reports only stated it was "atypical," which we took to mean benign (non-cancerous). The doctors told us the mole was nothing to worry about, and it was only removed as a preventive measure.

Now, at age fifteen, there was this lump located on the same side where the mole used to be but the lump was behind my ear. It didn't hurt or get in the way of anything, but it had been there since November and didn't seem to be going away. I just pretty much ignored it and didn't think it would be anything to worry about.

While my parents, Charlie and Cherie, were also excited I made it onto the junior varsity baseball team, my mom wasn't as laid-back as I was about the lump behind my ear. She's like that, though—a go-getter type who wants to fix things. It wasn't a surprise when she made an appointment with the doctor for me.

I didn't know it at the time, but that appointment would be the first inning—the first kick-off—of the most important game in life that I've ever played.

Cherie Rood

Any mother is happy when she sees that her child is happy. Trey is my firstborn. He's a pretty easygoing kid, the kind of boy everyone likes. He's got a sensitive and very kind personality, and doesn't get stressed easily. Trey started sports at a very young age. Even with his calm demeanor, he could be as competitive as the next player on any team.

When Trey made the junior varsity baseball team, I loved the way his eyes shone with enthusiasm as he shared the news with his dad and me.

The happiness didn't reflect pride, like thinking he was better than the rest. He was excited about getting the chance to become better at something. It was an honor for him to be chosen—something he (and his father and I) didn't expect his freshman year of high school. Trey put in great effort at try-outs. Although his making junior varsity was unexpected, it sure was a great "wow" moment for us as parents!

It's strange, though, how happiness can feel threatened in an instant, and how everything familiar can suddenly feel surreal. A room you know as well as your name becomes foggy and foreign when the unexpected enters. This was the atmosphere that invaded my home office one night, when Trey strolled in to talk about school, sports, and other things that take center stage in the mind of someone just shy of his fifteenth birthday. We had enjoyed many conversations in this room, but the comfortable familiarity of this night changed the second I noticed something lurking ominously behind Trey's right ear. Peering closer, I saw that it was a lump, maybe around half an inch in diameter.

"Trey, what is that?" I asked, trying not to sound, or feel, too alarmed.

"This?" He said, touching it with the casual nonchalance of a teenager who has better things to think about, like his new learner's permit, friends, and sports. "Just a little lump, I guess."

"How long has it been there?"

"A couple of months."

A couple of months? In my head, a million thoughts rushed in at once—all of them screaming cancer. Surely this wouldn't be the start of something bad. I tried to make all the thoughts go away, but I couldn't get my mind off it. I had to keep telling myself, it would be okay, stay positive, but there was just something in the back of my mind that wouldn't let it go.

I wanted to cover my ears, as if to block out the ceaseless chatter in my mind. I tried to hold the thoughts at bay, mentally denying the worst-case scenario. I went into survival mode and grounded myself in being proactive.

"We need to get that looked at," I said, forcing my voice to stay calm and steady despite the fear assaulting my thoughts. As I said the words, my mind was already rearranging my to-do list; investigating that lump moved straight to the top. I called Trey's pediatrician first thing in the morning, hoping this would prove to be nothing that a round of antibiotics wouldn't take care of. That's what I told Trey, for both his comfort and mine. After all, Trey had made JV baseball as a freshman! I was so proud of him; I couldn't let myself get down about this. Playing high school baseball would be a great privilege for him. I couldn't dampen his excitement with my motherly worries. I tried to focus on other things, and told myself it was just a swollen lymph node. It couldn't be cancer.

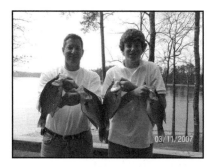

Charlie and Trey proud of the day's catch!

After Trey left my office, I made a beeline to the family room where my husband Charlie was watching television. As I passed through the hallway and kitchen into the family room, I was hyper-aware of the family pictures hanging on the walls, the backpacks and textbooks splayed out, and other bits and pieces that represented our active home and two teenage boys. This was our normal life—who we were as a family, and everything we knew and wanted life to be.

As I took in these everyday surroundings, though, my intuition—that "mother's instinct"—kicked in, as if warning that our lives were about to change. A chilling whisper as well as a burning affirmation, it just seemed to rise up from deep inside me, strong and unrelenting, no matter how hard I tried to shake it off.

I wasn't exactly sure how Charlie would respond to this discovery of Trey's lump. There had been a lot of cancer in Charlie's family, with Hodgkin's disease having taken his father at a young forty-five years of age. Most of our family had been healthy and blessed in many ways, but one of my greatest, longtime fears was that cancer would find its way to one of us. Yet, I had never allowed myself to think the disease would target one of my boys—and I definitely never imagined it was something any family member would face before adulthood.

"Charlie, Trey has this lump behind his ear," I said bluntly. "I'm calling the doctor tomorrow."

Charlie turned his attention away from the TV and toward me. He didn't ask me what I thought it was. Was he thinking it might be a virus? Strep throat? An injury? For a second, I wondered if he already knew the answer, the one I feared. He agreed that a check-up was in order, and that was the extent of our conversation.

Charlie's not one to wear his emotions on his sleeve. I realized that he might not be as alarmed as I was, so I decided to keep my feelings to myself for the time being. I felt like if I said out loud what I thought the lump was, it might actually be true. Scared and not knowing exactly where to start, I left the family room and just acted like this was going to be okay. Fear plagued my emotions. I knew I had to be strong. Surely nothing bad could come of this as long as I didn't think about it or say anything, right? I decided not to even tell many friends about it, so I wouldn't overanalyze the situation more than I already was. But deep down inside, it felt like a bomb had exploded.

Charlie Rood

Cancer wasn't the first thought that came to mind when Cherie told me about the lump behind our son's ear. I don't know why I didn't immediately start to worry about it, though. Cancer wasn't a stranger to my family. We not only lost my dad to it, but also his father and grandfather and one of his siblings. Everyone in the family had a different type of cancer, and none of the cancers were related. I wonder if there's something in the family DNA that makes us more susceptible. I've thought about that for a long time, but still didn't make an immediate connection between cancer and the lump behind Trey's ear.

Cherie made Trey's appointment with his pediatrician, who sent him to an ear-nose-throat (ENT) specialist after an initial examination. Because it was near Trey's parotid gland, which is a salivary gland that makes saliva, the ENT recommended the lump be removed. But first, he performed an aspiration biopsy, where a fine needle extracts a small amount of tissue from the parotid to test for the presence of malignant cells. We got the result fairly quickly, and it was benign, which was a relief. Following the biopsy on a separate visit, Trey required surgery to remove the lump. I still had lingering concerns, but pushed them aside. The doctor didn't seem worried, so I wasn't going to be either. He even said surgery could wait until after spring break, the first week of April. This was also around the middle of baseball season, and I knew Trey wouldn't be happy about his time on the field being interrupted.

Some people wondered why Cherie and I didn't just try to postpone the surgery until end of season, but we were too anxious. Even though the lump wasn't setting off any alarms with the doctor, it was still something that wasn't supposed to be there. We wanted it gone.

Cherie

Each year for spring break the boys and I took our traditional vacation, which most of the time was a cruise with friends Trey and his brother Wes went to school with or from the neighborhood. It had become a trip where the moms would take all the kids to keep it simple. So the dads all got their own break!

Spring break 2007 arrived, and Trey, Wes, and I boarded the ship. It was a week of balmy, Caribbean breezes, lots of sunshine, and me—a worried mother who just couldn't relax. Trey's surgery was scheduled just after our return home, and no one but me understood my big worries over a small lump. It was that foreboding intuition, and I just couldn't take a vacation from reality.

No matter where I was on the ship or the islands we visited, my intuition loomed over me like a dark storm cloud, ready to shower me with all sorts of life-threatening scenarios as I thought about Trey. He didn't seem concerned. Neither did Charlie or Wes! It appeared to be just me, even though I'm generally an upbeat person. I'm all about positivity, and I'm the first one in our family to find a way of combatting anything. Trey's lump, though, was a different story. Any good feelings I had following the aspiration biopsy were fading quickly. My very soul was seasick, churning with a nauseating uncertainty. Though I tried hard to enjoy the onboard fun and port excursions, I was only going through the motions.

We returned home from our week at sea and prepared for Trey's scheduled surgery. The closer the date came, the more pressure I felt building within me. I tried to stay busy and keep my mind off the bad stuff, but as soon as I thought the anxiety was conquered, it began to creep back in in the form of "what if?" What if Trey has cancer? A taunting answer would follow. It rattled me to the core: This is going to happen.

The lump was removed, followed by days of waiting for results. These were some of the longest hours of my life. The seemingly slow movement of time nearly put me over the edge. I desperately wanted answers, but was also terrified at the thought of them. Even though my cell phone never left my side, I was constantly checking it to make sure I hadn't missed any messages from the ENT doctor. I called his office day after day to see if the pathology report was in, but was always given the same frustrating answer: not yet.

I tried to subdue my anxiety and threw myself into my sales job, which allowed me to get out of the house, making calls and visits with clients. Yet, it didn't make the phone ring any sooner, and I needed that phone to ring. Good or bad, whatever news waited on the other end was news that would impact my family, especially Trey. It would decide if our lives continued as normal, or if they would be completely and forever changed. I couldn't help but feel like the waiting game was exceptionally cruel. Mostly, I hated the knowledge that my family's fate was pending and that I was powerless to speed up test results. I just needed to know: Was Trey okay or not?

It was April 12, 2007, when the call came in. I will forever remember exactly where I was—in my car on my way home from work, about three miles from the house. The ENT doctor called to deliver the word we had hoped and prayed we wouldn't hear: Malignant.

"Malignant . . . what?" I asked.

It's a word that never precedes good news, but sometimes it's quickly followed with assurance that the prognosis is hopeful, even in more advanced stages. You don't hear that, though, when the malignant cancer is melanoma.

For someone who, deep down, had sensed for a while that something was seriously wrong, I immediately sought comfort through my denial.

"No way," I argued. "This is not real. What about the clean biopsy and those benign cells?"

"Melanoma can hide in biopsies," the doctor explained. This is the problem with biopsies made by aspiration, we learned. The doctor inserts a needle into a suspicious lump and withdraws whatever is in the vicinity of its point. If healthy cells happen to be in that specific area, then that's what gets retrieved and analyzed. If malignant cells are in that area, then that's what gets extracted for analysis.

More questions flooded my brain, so many that I could barely grasp one before another charged up on its heels. I was a stranger to the world of melanoma, but listened amid a growing cold sweat as this doctor explained that it's one of the deadliest types of cancer there is. It's very treatable when caught early, but Trey's didn't appear to have been caught early enough. Though they had not yet determined just how progressed his cancer was, the biopsy indicated that the best we could hope for was stage III—meaning it had spread to nearby lymph nodes and areas of the skin, but not to vital organs. The bottom line: It was serious, life-threatening, and any treatment options would be aggressive.

I had one hand on the steering wheel and the other gripping my cell phone. I'm not sure how I processed the news without careening right off the winding back roads that led into my neighborhood. The landscape outside my car window was a combination of quiet countryside and residential community, but now it all appeared a blur of colors, lacking any defining lines, just a distorted fuzzy picture—a good analogy for how our lives suddenly seemed.

My son had melanoma. My seemingly healthy, athletic, fifteen-year-old son had melanoma—an aggressive, merciless form of cancer that didn't care how young he was, how much living he still had to do, and how much I loved him. It didn't care, and even worse, it felt bigger than all of us.

What I remember next is fumbling with my cell phone as I quickly called Charlie's office. I don't really recall how I told him. I just remember he said he was leaving work that very minute.

Charlie

How could they have screwed that up?! That was my first thought after Cherie called me about the results. Based on what we were led to think earlier from a "clean" biopsy and surgery performed under no big rush, I was in a state of shock. The shock, though, wasn't deep enough to withhold the anger over what felt like gross misinformation. This was our son they were talking about, a human being—not a car or a boat the mechanic tells you needs a little more work than you originally estimated.

It was incredible how quickly life shifted. In one phone call, I went from thinking about Wes's lacrosse game that night to figuring out how to tell Trey he had cancer.

Cherie was devastated, as any mother would be, fighting to be strong and hold back her emotions, but unable to. How was a mother to cope, or imagine her fifteen-year-old taking this kind of news? How did she fear this might affect him? I could feel the incredible pain she felt for him, and I knew she couldn't imagine being the one to face him and deliver the absurdity of this devastating news.

She had also been on the Internet, where Google searches called up an overwhelming mountain of information, none of it encouraging. I mean, none of it. Whether stage III or stage IV, our son would be facing a brutal monster that acts fast—and it usually came out the winner.

Men have moments with their sons that they never forget. From the day they're born, we look forward to such moments, imagining those things that guys bond over—the glory of reeling in a big fish together, the mutual thumbs-up when he's just made a great play on the field, the pat on the back when he tells you he just might love that girl he's been seeing. What you never imagine is a father-son moment forever marked by the word "cancer." Despite having lived my whole life in a family that had heard it a lot, I was no more prepared for it than someone who's never experienced it with a loved one.

People have asked me how I did it: How did I break the news? What did I say? How did I say it? How do you tell your child he has cancer? There's really no good way you can say something like that to anyone, much less a teenage boy who thinks the toughest battle he's got in the immediate future is the rigors of spring football practice.

Our game would be different, our season tougher—and that's what I told Trey. "There's been a change of plans." That day was the moment that changed the game plan forever.

Chapter Two

Trey

When my dad told me there was going to be "a change of plans," I really wasn't sure what he was talking about. I hoped he wasn't talking about canceling any summer plans to go to Sea Island, Georgia! That's where we spent time every summer with the Foster family, who are some of my parents' best friends. I've always loved it there. Instead, the change Dad was talking about was something much bigger than life itself, something I would live with forever.

It was Thursday, April 12, 2007. We were on the deck behind our house when Dad broke the news. "The doctors say you have cancer, Trey."

My dad is not a man of many words. He gets to the point quickly. But cancer . . . was this for real? Wow. I just stared. I'm not sure how long that empty state of mind lasted, but the first thought I remember having was, "Why would God do this to me?"

I stared out beyond the backyard for a while, seeing things that looked exactly the way they had moments before this revelation. Although they appeared to be the same . . . I wasn't. I wasn't the same. Considering I had cancer that had already hit at least stage III, I guessed I really hadn't been the same for a while. Dad explained to me the tumor had been tested, and the results were not good. I immediately thought that maybe they were wrong. Maybe the tumor was just an isolated thing and there wouldn't be much to it. I had no idea what I was getting into as a new cancer patient and how it would end up being the toughest play of my life to defeat.

I think, from the moment it sunk in, I knew one thing: I didn't want anything to set me apart from normal teenagers. I couldn't let cancer get in my way; I wanted to keep doing all the things I normally did—sports, practice, summer golf, beach trips, and wakeboarding. Cancer couldn't take those away! Maybe that's why one of the first things I asked my dad was if I could still play football, and if we would still go to Sea Island. Dad couldn't give me definitive answers to either question, but promised that he and Mom were going to do everything in their power to help me fight this thing.

As far as thoughts on the whole of my life at that point, I wasn't concerned about it the way some might think. Dying wasn't really on my schedule, and I knew I had some work to do to keep it that way. I'm not the type of person that dwells on any one thing—not even something this big, believe it or not. I knew right away I had to accept that I had cancer. There wasn't any time to figure it out, but I knew God would walk me through this and I would be okay.

Football had taught me that you never give up. You fight like every play is just as important as the biggest play you could ever experience. *I can handle this*, I thought. Cancer could be the biggest play of my life, but I wasn't going to let it win. It never occurred to me that I wouldn't win. My mind was already set, and I just wanted someone to let me know what I needed to do. It is what it is, I thought, and time to move on.

"All right," I told my dad. "What's next?"

Cherie

I hid in my home office while Charlie broke the news to Trey. I didn't want Trey to see me cry, didn't want him to see that the mother who could always take the bull by the horns was actually terrified. Dear God, it sounded so relentless. Would I even have the strength to help Trey fight this? Waiting for Charlie to give Trey the devastating news, I already felt like every part of my being was whipped and beaten down. I learned that night what it really feels like to have a broken heart—whether it's shattered like glass, slowly ripped to shreds or quickly snapped in two, it opens up an agony both emotional and physical. It hurt just as much to breathe and swallow as it did to think and wonder. Crying huddled in my office, I had never felt so spirit-wounded and vulnerable to fear and despair, both of which were ready to engulf the space in my heart that held peace and dreams. Did I have any life experience to help Trey power through this? I didn't think so. Did I have anything within me to do it, anyway? I could only pray I would.

Charlie assured me that Trey reacted to the news pretty well. That was a relief, and something I wasn't surprised to hear. I really wasn't. It's often said that the person most impacted by a serious disease is the one who handles it best. Everybody else feels helpless, because how do you comfort? How do you stay strong with this thing hurting your loved one? Trey was also young, with an invincible outlook many kids feel in their innocence. Maybe it helped convince him that this was something he could beat. Mainly, though, I think it's just that Trey had always carried a winner's attitude. He'd never backed down from adversity before. Granted, his hands-on experience with this approach was mostly lived on the athletic field, but it was still a reflection of his resolve to outrun and outplay any opponent. Now, as he prepared to take on this very different opponent—by far, the biggest one to date—I knew I had to be strong and present. I had to be at the game with him, but instead of watching from the sidelines, I needed to be right on the field.

As I listened to Charlie recount his conversation with Trey, I gathered myself, discarding the poor-pitiful-me heap of tears I had collapsed into. It was Trey's strength that lifted me. It was time for him to see that Mom was going to be okay.

"I can do this," I vowed as I headed toward Trey's room. "I will do this."

But . . . do what? We felt lost as to which way to turn. There were options, but which one was best? Our wait to see the doctors felt ridiculously long, given the serious nature of Trey's diagnosis. I always feel better when I'm being proactive, but I didn't know where to put my energies or how to quickly get my son the optimum care.

Frustrations aside, all around us angels arose in the form of family, friends, and community members, stepping forward to ease our burdens and offer support in a wide range of ways. Among them were our friends Brad and Marie Foster, who, at the time, served on the board at Children's

Healthcare of Atlanta Foundation. When they contacted the director of the Aflac Cancer Center (part of Children's Health Care) about us, and received the affirmation that we would be properly guided along the road ahead, I knew that something was answering our prayers for clarity. We frantically researched, called, and begged to speak with a doctor there. It was Dr. Lewis Rapkin who followed up with a callback. Charlie and I spoke to him for a while. He reassured us that we were coming to the right place, and that Trey wasn't the first melanoma patient they had treated or seen.

We were jumpy and anxious, almost overwhelmed, by the anticipation of meeting Dr. Rapkin. Waiting for our appointment was so difficult because we were starving for information about what was ahead. At the moment, we weren't doing anything but waiting. No action was being taken. No plan was in the works. We wanted to be proactive, to feel like and know that we were doing something—anything—to fight this monster. The appointment with Dr. Rapkin couldn't arrive soon enough. What we wanted to hear was that he knew how to make Trey's cancer go away, that he would map out a plan to put this dreadful disease behind us.

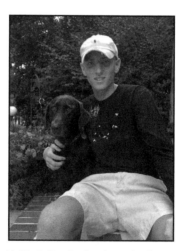

Trey with Ms. Bailey, the chocolate Labrador we got him
shortly after his melanoma diagnosis.

Despite our eagerness to meet Dr. Rapkin, walking through those sliding glass doors at the Aflac Cancer Center was harrowing. It burns like salt in a raw wound to walk into a pediatric institution and face children whose lives have been suspended by diseases, medications, and treatments that many can't even pronounce, much less understand. It's devastating to truly comprehend that one of your own children is now a member of that world.

Yet another angel appeared within minutes of our arrival. Her name was Robin Pitts, and she was the mother of a young lady Trey had dated. I didn't know she worked at the cancer center, but there she was, at precisely the moment we valued a familiar face. She walked us through an introduction to the center.

We spent an intense, three-hour consultation with Dr. Rapkin. Because Trey was a pediatric patient with an adult disease, physicians from the nearby Winship Cancer Institute of Emory University were also called in to consult. Both facilities are among the top in the nation, and we felt good about the doctors' interest in our case. All of the medical professionals spoke openly in front of Trey, and confirmed that we were likely faced with stage III melanoma, best-case scenario. I was determined not to let myself think beyond that.

My vow to see this through changed from "I can do this" to "We can do this," as it was clearly affirmed that we were not alone. We were taking this journey together. It was our life now. It had become part of who we were, and it was time to get a new game plan in motion.

A lymph node dissection would tell us if the cancer was confined to the original site, or if it had strayed to Trey's lymph nodes. First, Trey underwent a full body positron emission tomography (PET) scan at Emory/Winship (where all of his scans would be done) to see if the cancer had spread to his lungs, brain, or any other organs. If the scan came back positive, there would be no reason to go forward with the surgery. We would know that the cancer was stage IV, the very worst it could be, and that the disease was at an even greater advantage.

It had only been a couple of days since Trey's scan, which had not been a fun experience for him. At the time, Emory/Winship really didn't have a great "warm and fuzzy" facility to go to for a PET scan. It felt like we were in a dungeon. Maybe we felt like that since Trey and I were fighting the fact that cancer was going to be a part of our lives, and anything associated with it was not somewhere we wanted to be.

I was sitting in the dentist's chair when my cell phone rang. Dr. Rapkin's name flashed across the screen. This was it—the call I had been dreading, mixed with anxiety and prayers that it would bring good news. It felt like forever waiting for Dr. Rapkin's call. So many emotions were attached to this call, and whatever answers it delivered would directly impact Trey's very life and our family's future.

I'm not sure there are adequate words to describe what I felt, sitting in the dentist's chair, listening to Dr. Rapkin reveal that the PET scan was negative and there were no traces of cancer in any of Trey's organs. All the fears and torturous what ifs of stage IV cancer suddenly washed away in tears of relief and happiness. God was giving us more time to figure out this deadly monster. We were gratefully cleared to go in for the lymph node dissection surgery at Egleston Children's Hospital on the Emory University campus. Now we just had to hope and pray that the results from that would be as clean as the PET scan.

Trey

I was determined to keep my life as normal as possible and not stand out, but the game plan caused some havoc with that. For one thing, I wouldn't finish my freshman year of high school at South Forsyth with my friends. Instead, I spent the last month of that year getting hospital/homebound services; tutors brought assignments to our house and I completed a lot of my homework online. Of course, baseball ended early for me. Summer football workouts weren't looking too likely, either. Baseball wasn't so important, but I really didn't want to miss football; it was my passion.

To do the lymph node dissection, doctors cut close behind my ear (where the tumor had been removed) and down along the right side of my neck, up to the center of my throat. The incision branded me with a horseshoe mark for a while—just what all teenagers want when they want to blend in with everyone else!

The operation took four hours. I guess they were long hours for my parents and grandma, who drove in from Kentucky. I later learned that Clay Scroggins and Kevin Ragsdale, leaders from my small bible study group at Browns Bridge Community Church, showed up unexpectedly at the hospital. My mom wasn't even sure who they were at first—a couple of young guys in jeans and casual shirts. They stayed with my parents for a long time, praying and extending so much support. I just thought that was so cool. We lived in Cumming, and Clay and Kevin drove an hour down to Atlanta . . . just for me? It meant so much to us.

So many things meant a lot to me in those early days, maybe because it was my first real understanding of how much it matters to have good people in your life. As word got out about what was going on with my illness, people came together to support and encourage our family. One of the first things to happen was a prayer vigil held at the home of our good family friends, the Smiths. A pastor of Midway Community Church, Dean Rop, presided over a prayer vigil for me. Melissa Smith organized it and the event brought out a ton of kids and adults, all there just to pray . . . for me. It was amazing. I couldn't believe how many of my friends were there—there for me. Ben Sasser was another good friend of mine who I'd played with on many baseball and football teams for years. He had hundreds of blue wristbands made that were imprinted with a cross, a football, and the words, "Pray for Trey." When I found out that a lot of kids at school, and practically every guy on the football team, were wearing one of the wristbands, my mind was blown.

I was never alone, because friends were around me all the time. I'm not sure what I would have done if they hadn't been. I think their presence had something to do with why I didn't get it when people worried about me becoming depressed. Depression seemed to be a big concern for the adults, but really—it never crossed my mind. I worried about my brother

Wes, though. How was all of this hitting him? When you learn that an older person in your family has cancer, it isn't often your very own sibling.

Wes Rood

I was only in seventh grade when my brother got his diagnosis. I had just turned thirteen, and at the time, didn't really understand all the things suddenly going on in and around our family. I knew Trey had cancer, but didn't get how serious it was or how deadly it could be.

Trey and I have had our fights, just like all brothers do, but there was never a time we weren't close. I guess I was taking my cues from him on the cancer. Whatever exactly was going on with it, he wasn't letting it keep him down. His optimistic attitude influenced mine right from the start.

There were so many people supporting him and all of us. Trey's friends were everywhere and acting normal whenever they were around him. None of them changed their personalities, and that was comforting to see. It made me feel like everything would be okay.

The "Pray for Trey" wristbands were a huge hit with everyone. I guess the football players at South High were the first people to start wearing them. After that, they took off like wildfire. Even the kids at my school at Vickery Creek were wearing them. I saw them in class, the locker room, the hallways. In a way, it was strange to see so many people, even many I didn't know, wearing these blue bands for something so personal to my family. Mostly, though, it was great to see all the people pulling for us.

I've been wearing my wristband since the first day they came out. I've had to replace a few over the years, but I've never missed a day of wearing one. It never comes off, not even in the shower.

Charlie

I was dumbfounded by the outpouring of support. It blew my mind. Every time someone did something nice for us, I thought, "Wow, a lot of people like Cherie," or "That was for Trey, Cherie, and Wes." I couldn't imagine why anyone would want to do such nice things for me.

It was very humbling to be on the receiving end of this type of kindness from people who expected nothing in return. They just wanted to help. Period. We had so much food being brought over that we actually had to start asking people to reschedule their plans for delivery. We couldn't eat it fast enough—and with three males living in the house, that tells you something!

It took a couple of weeks before we knew the results of Trey's lymph node dissection, and waiting proved to be one of the hardest parts for me. Finally, after praying that no further melanoma would be found, we learned that there were traces of it in two lymph nodes. He was in stage III C of the disease, just barely under stage IV, which is as bad as it gets.

Just as he did after the first surgery, Trey wanted to know what he needed to do and what the plan was. Well, it would be intense, just as we were warned. It would start with infusions of interferon, which is a natural protein made by the immune system. Trey would get the infusions every day for twenty days, followed by eleven months of interferon injections given three times a week from home. Interferon has been shown to promote the growth of two white blood cells, T and B lymphocytes, to increase immunities and stop cancer from spreading.

That was the plan that we entrusted the Aflac and Emory/Winship doctors with to save our son's life.

Cherie

The revelation that there were traces of melanoma in Trey's lymph nodes knocked me off the pillar of hope I had been clinging to. I had prayed that maybe, just maybe, the doctors would find clear nodes and their suspicions about Trey's cancer stage would be wrong. The doctor explained there were only two affected lymph nodes out of the many that had been removed during surgery, but this news proved to me that Trey's melanoma had its own agenda. It's really happening, and this confirms it. My son has a deadly form of cancer.

"But Cherie, it was only found in two nodes," my mother said, trying to encourage me.

The small number of lymph nodes involved didn't matter to me. The cancer had made it to Trey's lymph nodes. It wasn't confined to the original site. Whether it was in two nodes or two hundred, I felt like the book had been thrown at us.

As strange as this may sound at first, I also internally struggled with all the support our family was receiving from the community. It was awesome and I was touched, but I was concerned that the ongoing reminders would start to work against Trey's winning attitude, and I was all about keeping him focused on beating this disease. Part of me feared it might drive home just how serious this all was, and reinforce the life-or-death battle we were facing. I wondered if it could backfire and have a negative effect on Trey's outlook.

The number of kids wearing the "Pray for Trey" wristbands, though, was astonishing. They rallied around Trey. I came to see that the moral support was playing a huge role in keeping his attitude on track, and it was too important. In hindsight, I see that our road would have been more unbearable without it. Our good friend and neighbor, Dodi Mace, and her daughter Cailin, Trey's childhood friend, set up a "Pray for Trey" Facebook page. It quickly became a meeting place to share updates, needs, and post those uplifting words of encouragement.

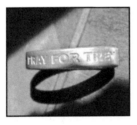

The "Pray for Trey" wristband.

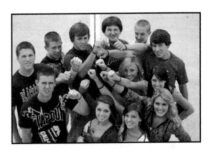

Many students and folks in the community
sporting the "Pray for Trey" wristbands to
show their support.

Trey's interferon infusions were heavy and intense. The process took six hours a day for those first twenty days in May and June. With weekend breaks, this was prime "lake time" in Trey's book, but a port in his arm meant that his love for wakeboarding and waterskiing were going to have to wait awhile. Trey loves Lake Lanier, which is only fifteen minutes from our house. It's been a big part of Charlie's family since before he was born, and holds many great memories. Trey still went to the lake when he felt up to it and watched his friends swim, never seeming to begrudge them their summer fun. Quiet and non-complaining, he just seemed to accept that he had a disease that didn't discriminate. It didn't matter to melanoma that Trey was a kid who wanted to be in the water.

While Trey was accepting of his melanoma, he wasn't defined by it. To him, it was something he didn't plan on dealing with for the rest of his life. His goal was to get well, beat it, and move on. It was a temporary intruder, and the interferon treatment was his best chance of removing any evidence of it from his body.

Trey was willing to do whatever it took to beat melanoma, even though the interferon had side effects. Flu-like symptoms were the norm during treatments and infusions. He would often develop a fever, body aches, and chills to the point of shaking uncontrollably. Thankfully, the symptoms didn't linger for long periods of time, so when he was able to switch over to shots three times a week, we timed them so that he could eat dinner before the symptoms kicked in. After a couple of hours, he usually fell asleep and woke up in the morning feeling better.

Overall, Trey's treatment was going well and we focused on keeping him and every member of his large support team optimistic. Even with my own determination to stay positive, though, I still found myself crying a lot. Sometimes it was enough to make me wonder if I was a bottomless well of tears. The jags could be triggered by anything and always left me wondering when, if ever, they would stop. Other times I was gripped by that wrenching feeling that my heart was literally, physically breaking. At such times, I was especially thankful for the good friends who surrounded me. I remember telling my dear friend and neighbor, Dee Todd, that I wasn't sure I would ever get past my broken heart, that I would ever get past this cross my was family was forced to carry.

Despite our growing familiarity with the Aflac Cancer Center, and our easy transition into home treatments, it was very hard for me to accept this as our life's reality. I had a child with cancer, and that was something I would cope with for the rest of my days. Even if Trey were cured, there would still be lifelong follow-ups. There would be hold-your-breath-and-wait-and-see scares every time some unusual symptom popped up, even if it was one that could be attributed to numerous non–life-threatening ailments. I struggled with the cold truth of our situation. I often found myself staring longingly after neighbors whose children were untouched by cancer, who played and went to school with nothing nearly as pressing on their minds. I grieved deeply for the normal life we had known before, and wished again for the less challenging pace of our lives then.

We weren't that family anymore. I knew we all had to accept and live life where we were, define a new normal, and walk in the world of cancer with Trey. Though private breakdowns were bound to happen, and stress would sometimes get the better of us, I remained committed to Trey's exposure to as much hope, encouragement, and positivity as we could muster. There actually proved to be a lot of it, so while we were not a typical family, we were definitely a positive one.

Trey wasn't a typical patient at the Aflac Cancer Center, either. Melanoma is more of an adult cancer. Even though Aflac had treated other melanoma pediatric patients, it just wasn't seen as frequently as many of the other childhood cancers. Trey was only considered half-child. The other half was adult, and that's the side melanoma usually favors. After all, he was a six-foot-three teenager. This made Trey a rare and slightly foreign case for the Aflac nurses who weren't used to administering interferon to patients. Though they were excellent nurses, their unfamiliarity with Trey's specific cancer-fighting potion did not do a lot for my comfort level. Trey's unique half-and-half position only added to the feeling of limbo that often goes along with cancer treatment.

Trey, too, was not in his comfort zone at Aflac. He wouldn't have been at any facility like it. During the daily visits, we noticed almost immediately that he kept to himself and chose not to interact with other patients or their families. He was older than most of the other patients, but it was also evident that Trey wanted no part of the cancer world. It was a sign that he saw his ordeal as a passing season that he wanted to put behind him as quickly as possible. Social workers tried to get him involved with patient activities, but he just wasn't on board.

Trey

People talk a lot about how young fifteen is to be diagnosed with cancer. It is, but I'm far from the youngest person to get that kind of news. There were people much younger than me at the Aflac Cancer Center, and even some little kids in my own community dealing with it.

It bothered me to see someone that young with cancer. You feel really bad for those kids, and think how wrong and unfair it is that they aren't living a normal life for their age. When I saw a really young kid with cancer, I kind of knew what older people thought when they saw me.

I was determined to get back to a normal life. I'm glad my parents decided to "live life as we were" before I got sick. They didn't stop me from doing what I felt like I could do, as long as my doctors said it wouldn't be dangerous or set me back.

The first twenty days of interferon infusions felt like forever, though. The daily trips to the hospital and the long hours spent there got real old, real fast, but we slowly counted them down. In fact, the whole summer was an anxious time for me, because I was learning what to expect regarding the side effects. I didn't always know from day to day how I was going to feel. When we transitioned to the three-shots-a-week routine, I at least got to take them at home and deal with the side effects more comfortably. They were quick—not a six-hour deal. We started timing them around my activities and dinnertime, which helped, though there were some days when the side effects got their punches in.

There was one thing I wanted to do more than anything that summer:

go to football practice. It became my motivation to fight melanoma, as well as my way of escaping for a while. Even on the days I didn't really feel like going, I still went to practice. It was worth any effort, because I felt normal when I put on my gear and stepped onto the field with all the other guys. Stepping onto the football field was the only time I didn't really think about melanoma.

Besides football practice being an escape, it was also a chance to check out the facilities of the brand new high school opening in my community. Along with most of my friends, I would be leaving South Forsyth to start my sophomore year at West Forsyth, which was just a couple of miles from my house. A lot of guys were excited to be part of a new football program they could help build from the ground floor.

The head coach was Frank Hepler. He was moving up from southern Florida, where he'd been coaching high school football for a long time. He had an amazing track record for wins and getting his players recruited by colleges, so everyone was looking forward to meeting him. He'd been head coach at one high school for many years. Then he had stepped down to assistant coach for a couple of years and be more available while his wife, a breast cancer survivor, was getting treatment.

Moving to West Forsyth, Georgia, was obviously a big decision for Coach Hepler. He not only uprooted his family, but also asked some of his Florida coaching staff to consider making the move too. After he accepted the job offer from West Forsyth, but before he'd officially moved, he visited the area to have a big meeting with the players' parents. That was when a kind of cool story started getting around.

It turns out that, while he was deciding whether to take the job, he heard from someone in the community about "this guy named Trey," a high school football player who had cancer. He learned about how the community and the future West Forsyth football team were coming together to "Pray for Trey" and offer all kinds of support to the family. Coach Hepler said that was when he told his wife that our community and our team was where they needed to be.

Chapter Three

Trey

My sophomore year of high school started, and the interferon treatments continued through most of it. I lost fifteen pounds that year, mainly because my appetite wasn't steady. That was unusual during football season, when most guys are eating a lot more. Again, we tried to plan the shots around my activities and school hours, but the side effects still sometimes got to me.

Unlike a lot of people getting treated for cancer, though, I didn't lose my hair. It got kind of brittle and even turned a little orange, but there really weren't any drastic changes in my physical appearance. I did everything I could to keep living like the average teenager.

Football was great that year. I think a lot of people expected us to have a terrible season because we were a brand new program. It's true that it often takes new teams a few years to get established and start winning, but we came out strong and had a 9-1 season. I loved wearing my "5" jersey and starting as free safety. Plus, everyone gave me a lot of moral support mainly by just treating me like every other player on the team. One difference, though, was that all my teammates kept wearing the "Pray for Trey" wristbands. Players from other schools started wearing them as well. That says a lot about the kind of community I lived in. We went after each other on the field, but off the field, everyone was saying, "Man, I hope you're going to be okay."

I never thought I wouldn't be okay. My plan from the start was to beat melanoma. I really didn't think the fight would ever get worse than what was going on at the time. Facing almost a year of interferon shots wasn't what

I'd call "normal living," but they'd be finished before my junior year of high school, which is an important one for anybody hoping to get recruited to play college football. I had full-body PET scans every three months during the interferon treatments. They were just part of the agenda, and something I had to do to put melanoma behind me.

Cherie

That fall, Trey had more PET scans at Emory/Winship in Atlanta. Thanks to a friend, Noreen Johnson, who was in medical sales and understood the process, I had someone who could answer my questions in layman's terms. Again, another angel to make this mother's walk a little easier. The more informed I was about what was being done for my son, the more adequate I felt in making decisions about his care. I couldn't just nod my head and go along with things I didn't understand. After all, this was Trey's life. There couldn't be any bad calls. I had to be assured that he was receiving the most accurate testing and the most successful treatments. Then, there was the period of waiting for results.

We were on the prayer lists of many churches, Bible study groups, and individuals. My specific prayer request was that the last of Trey's cancer had been confined to the lymph nodes that were removed during his second surgery, and that no cells had escaped to take up hiding elsewhere in his body. I tried to keep everyone steering forward. I stayed busy with everyday aspects of living, maybe even to the point of driving everyone around me crazy, as I found one more thing in the house to fix, clean, or get organized. The littlest task could become a big project as I marched ahead, intent on keeping my mind and my hands occupied. Every time a task was completed, I checked it off my list and enjoyed the sense of accomplishment. No grass grew under my feet before I found another project to take the place of the one we had just finished. "No rest for the weary" might have been a good motto for our house. I couldn't rest, fearing it would be idle time that might invite fears of cancer to come inside and dwell.

I also immersed myself in work, but quickly found myself relating to clients and customers in a new way. People I usually only discussed business with were putting it aside and taking the time to ask me how Trey was doing. I was so touched by the concern shown by people who didn't know me outside of the professional realm. As I shared some of our experiences with them, many would in turn tell me about a struggle they had faced or were currently dealing with. Suddenly, we were connecting in a deeper and more personal way. It hit home that we just don't always know what makes up a person's life story, and that we might be very surprised at how much we have in common.

No matter how busy I managed to keep myself, the dates of Trey's PET scans were the most important ones on the calendar. There was no way to forget that cancer had barged into our world, and the PET scans were the assurance that treatment had succeeded in chasing it away. Every time Trey had one, I held my breath, awaiting the doctor's call. I always sighed with relief when the scans showed clean results and gave us license to relax somewhat for another three months.

The Friday night lights of football season were exciting. We watched Trey play his first year at a brand new high school, while Wes played his final year in middle school. Trey lived to be on the field. He was well enough to play in the inaugural season opener, where he made the first interception in the history of West Forsyth football. He also made the first baseball team the following spring, and was honored with a coach's award from head coach Byron Orr. Any confidence that melanoma tried to snatch from Trey was coming back with a vengeance through his involvement with sports.

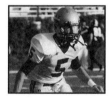

Trey where he was happiest—on the football field in 2007.

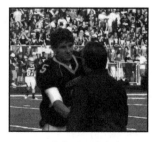

Trey shakes hands before interviewing with NBC affiliate sports broadcaster Randy Waters.

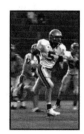

Trey on the field.

It wasn't just his actual performance on the field that built him up, though. It was the circle of support from his teammates and coaches at West Forsyth, as well as a former football coach from his playing days in middle school. Mark Taylor had been an assistant coach during Trey's years at Vickery Creek, but was actually leading the team as Wes's head coach. He also helped the new high school as a weight training instructor. In the process, he became a mentor for Trey by always encouraging him to play.

While I suppose there are some who think the coaches should have excused Trey from athletics, doing that could have been one of the worst moves ever. They certainly never pushed him to go past what he felt able to do, but the fact that they encouraged him to get out there did wonders for Trey's self-esteem. It proved to Trey that they believed in him and didn't think the cancer diminished him in any way. This, I believe, had a lot to do with why Trey's positive attitude never seemed to waver.

Trey's optimistic outlook fed my own attitude well. We were thrilled to count down to his final interferon shot, which came in late April of 2008. Another PET scan would follow it. We knew it wouldn't be Trey's last scan by any means. Many more would follow to confirm the melanoma had not returned, but the first scan to follow that last shot would feel like a huge milestone if it came back clean.

The report that the scan was exactly as we had prayed was like getting a pass to cross the bridge back into familiar territory. For the better part of a year, we had all been navigating unknown streets and following maps drawn by others. Now we were returning to a life without treatments and side effects— hopefully, one that would stay cancer-free.

Charlie

Word spread fast that Trey's melanoma was under control, but the doctors never used the word "remission" nor told us there was no evidence of disease. Trey, his mom, and I took what we could get, though, which thankfully happened to be that no cancer was lighting up on Trey's PET scan results. Go God!

I never considered Trey to be in an actual remission, either. My family's history with cancer isn't what colored my thoughts on that, though. It was because I knew there was a possibility that melanoma was still floating around somewhere in his body and could rear its ugly head again. Depending on which source you're reading, some say there is up to a seventy percent chance stage III melanoma will come back as stage IV. I was hopeful we were done with it, but never accepted it as a certainty.

I didn't dwell on it, though. That summer was like the ones we had enjoyed for years. Trey was sixteen now and didn't have any limitations from the melanoma, so he, Wes, and a lot of friends used the family lake house on Lake Lanier every chance they got. We also fished and played golf. With Wes headed into his freshman year of high school, both boys had football workouts and practices at West Forsyth. Our lives seemed a lot more on par for a family with two teenage sons, and much more like what we always imagined those years would be like. With treatment behind him, Trey quickly started putting some weight back on.

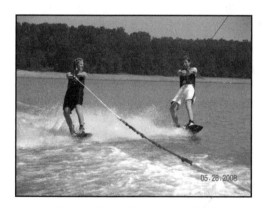

From left to right: Wes and Trey wakeboarding in easier times.

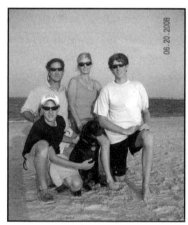

Sea Island on the Georgia coast during the summer of 2008.

He was discovering a new interest, too: getting involved with programs to raise money for cancer research or help cover the medical expenses of patients in treatment. At the end of June, he and Cherie both took part in our local community drive to support the Noreen O'Neill Foundation for Melanoma Research and the Wistar Institute, both headquartered in Philadelphia. There was another family in our community who had also been hit with melanoma. They organized the event called "Running for Cover," a 5K run/1-mile walk.

It was inspiring to see Trey become proactive in this type of service work. Earlier, he had wanted to distance himself from everything he could that was related to cancer, but now he was making his contribution to bringing the disease down. His involvement with the benefit was featured in the first newspaper article to really give a good overview of his own personal experience. That was published June 25, 2008, by the *Forsyth County News*: "Tackling a Disease; Local Athlete Kicks Cancer, Helps Fights for Cure" written by sports writer BJ Corbitt.

Trey's potential for earning a college football scholarship was looking good. During his junior season, scouts and coaches from Georgia Southern University, Furman University, and the University of West Georgia were all showing interest in recruiting him. Off the field, Trey is pretty quiet and a little on the shy side, but the *Atlanta Journal-Constitution* described him as "an electrifying player." He went into the year completely healthy at six-foot-three, and his weight ranging from a hundred and eighty to a hundred and eighty-eight pounds. Cherie and I watched proudly from the stands as he led the West Forsyth Wolverines in defense interceptions and ranked second in the number of tackles made. There was nothing shy about him on the gridiron. Later in the season, he was named to the 2008 All-County Team and to All Region Team.

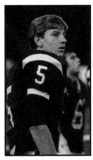

Trey's dreams of playing college football were looking a little closer to reality during his junior year at West Forsyth.

I was getting into a comfort zone with the way life was going. In the winter of 2009, we took the boys skiing and snowboarding in Colorado, which is something they both love as much as they do waterskiing and wakeboarding in the summer. Nobody who looked at Trey or watched him on the slopes would ever imagine this tall, lanky kid had battled something as life-threatening as stage III melanoma. Even people who knew him and his story well sometimes had a hard time remembering it, despite it only having been in the past year.

That spring, Trey went to classes as usual and he went to the junior-senior prom. In June, he went in for another PET scan . . . Cherie sat down at the computer and updated the "Pray for Trey" Facebook page.

Posted on June 18, 2009 at 2:17 p.m.:

"Trey's PET scan didn't go so well this time . . . appears to be a re-occurrence putting him in stage IV melanoma. Tests show the cancer has spread to his lungs and chest node area. Say a heavy prayer. We won't know any more for another week about what's next. Possibly a biopsy to confirm and then treatment. We can get through this and stay positive. We're going to keep Trey doing everything the same . . . God will work us through this!!"

I was shocked. Even though I'd never looked at that cancer-free year as a remission, the PET scans had been okay, and Trey looked and felt at the top of his game. I just couldn't believe how quickly it came back.

Trey

You've got to be kidding me. That's what I thought when I found out my cancer had come back, and right on the verge of my senior year of high school. I always knew it could come back. The thought crossed my mind every single day.

I just never thought it would come back. It was there, though, and I knew it was a lot worse this time.

Here we go again, I thought. At the time I thought it, I had no idea just how far we were going to go. All I knew was that I was going to do everything I could to keep playing football during my senior year. This was supposed to be any high school football player's big year, the one that would put me on the map. I wasn't going to miss it.

Chapter Four

Cherie

It wasn't just hard news to hear, it was hard to understand. For two years, and at regular intervals, Charlie and I had taken Trey to Emory/Winship for PET scans. They were always clean—and then suddenly they weren't. In a very short span of time, and with no warning, his melanoma was back with a vengeance.

I felt like we had been ambushed and sucker punched, just as Trey was about to be released and declared as cancer-free as he could get. I grieved for his youth being marred by the disease and for the senior year of high school that would not be the one he had hoped for. Just like the first time melanoma had entered our lives, I found that I could cry more tears than I knew my body could produce.

My thoughts couldn't stay in the dumps, though. I had to pick myself up and accept where we were in life, make the best of it, and tell myself to live one day at a time instead of thinking about all of the what ifs. I tried to grab onto Trey's attitude, where faith, hope, and determination were the rule. More "Pray for Trey" wristbands were ordered. I decided to commit harder than ever to believing what I was saying and writing updates. We can do this.

It was like deja vu that early June, as we returned to the Aflac Cancer Center where Emory/Winship was again consulting on Trey's case. Based on what they saw on Trey's most recent tests, doctors from the Winship Melanoma Tumor Board recommended that his left lung be removed.

Were they serious? The entire lung? I asked why they couldn't just remove the tumor. It was wrapped around a pulmonary artery leading from the heart, making removing only the tumor a very complicated and high-risk surgery. Its location was a game changer. With the news just seeming to get worse, we listened as doctors assured us they were following standard procedure for Trey's particular situation. Statistics showed that removing the cancer provided a better chance of survival or prolonged life.

Also, the standard treatment recommended after the lung was removed was the dreaded interleukin-2 treatment (IL-2), the one that saps your hope when you read about it. The treatment sounded so bad and seemed to offer so little upside that it would even work. We just weren't sure it was the right path to take. This time would be more intense than the interferon treatments were throughout his sophomore year. Over a period of six weeks, Trey would be admitted to the ICU at Scottish Rite, where the IL-2 was administered in three different rounds. Each round would keep him in the hospital for four to six days, sick enough from side effects that he would need maximum observation and care. The side effects could include intense, flu-like symptoms, high fevers, and violent chills, all of which could impact blood pressure, heart rate, and breathing. It just sounded awful.

When all was said and done, at the end of this treatment, minus one lung, Trey's chances of living to see another year were puny—something around five percent.

That, too, was a game changer, and reason to start thinking outside of the box. The question was: what else, if anything, could we do? Would this aggressive disease plow its way somewhere else in his body while we investigated other options?

Trey's doctors were waiting for a decision. With no other alternatives at the moment, we scheduled him to begin the IL-2 regimen in just a couple of weeks and met with the surgeon to start the pre-op process for his left lung removal. Lurking in the back of our minds, though, was a dark-clouded question: What if there was more cancer in his right lung that just hadn't shown up yet? What would we have really accomplished with all of this? Ultimately, we couldn't keep surgically removing Trey's cancer, only to find out a few months later that it had spread to his right lung. What then?

I snapped into complete survival mode, best described as tunnel vision intently and tightly focused on winning the hand we'd been dealt. I just didn't know what to focus on; I only knew we had to focus on pinpointing a solution—and fast.

Once home from the appointment with Trey's surgeon, I began researching other treatments. The news was dismal. Trey was not old enough to take part in any clinical trials being offered for melanoma in the United States. The minimum age was eighteen, according to the FDA's rules. It was yet another blow to us, so new at this. We quickly learned that once we stepped away from standard treatment options, we were on our own. Taking in to account that we were, once again, in the limbo state of facing an adult cancer in the pediatric world, the road ahead seemed bleak.

Trey was eight months shy of his eighteenth birthday. Most stage IV melanoma patients don't survive that long, and that filled me with despair. The more relaxed pace of Trey's junior year had quickly vanished, replaced with the daunting task of making phone calls around the country to various research centers and hospitals. I even looked beyond our own borders, researching medical news sites based in Germany, where promising treatments were taking place. Yet, they were a world away, and I had no idea if they would help Trey.

The next day, I joined some neighborhood women for an early morning walk, hopeful the summer air would clear my head as we briskly paced down the blocks. I walked the sidewalks my boys had taken their bikes on, passed lawns they had played front-yard football in, strolled past the driveways and basketball goals they had shot hoops into. Those days seemed like mere weeks ago, yet also like a million years ago. So much had changed. Life was nothing like I dreamed it would be, and everything I feared it could be.

On this morning, Noreen Johnson, my friend who had been so helpful early on during the PET scans, joined our walking group. Noreen and I weren't typically able to walk at the same time due to our work schedules, but as luck would have it, she was there that morning as I opened up to the group about all the scary stuff that was going on with Trey's recent relapse. I told them all about the research I was doing, and how we needed to consider everything and anything at that point. When I mentioned my interest in approved treatments Germany was using, Noreen responded.

"Well, isn't it ironic that this conversation came up today?" she asked. "My former brother-in-law is Dr. Rigdon Lentz, and he's doing oncology work in Germany."

Hope surged. I wanted to hear everything about this doctor, an American oncologist located in Prien am Chiemsee, Germany. She told me that Dr. Lentz ran a practice there where he offered a treatment called immunepheresis. Unlike chemotherapy and radiation treatments that weaken the entire body, this treatment claims to work with the body's natural immune system to destroy cancer cells. It first requires a venous catheter implant for the patient. In a process similar to dialysis, blood is then drawn from the catheter through a tubing system that feeds into a machine, which filters out inhibitors that block the immune system from fighting cancer. Removing these inhibitors empowers the immune system to attack cancer cells. The filtered blood is then routed back into the patient.

The study of immunepheresis claims to answer one of the most baffling questions about cancer: Why doesn't the patient's own immune system fight off and destroy cancer cells? Believing the culprit is the inhibitors in the blood, Dr. Lentz devoted years to research. He took his practice to Germany because of complications in getting the treatment approved in America.

It was a fascinating treatment, but also lengthy and expensive—most certainly one our insurance wouldn't cover. Yet, it boasted a possible thirty-five to fifty percent survival rate, which completely trumped the super low IL-2 survival rate.

Charlie

After the Aflac visit and hearing Trey's best, standard option at home, I was all for a trip to Germany to see if he was a good candidate for immunepheresis. Yet, I was also apprehensive, not knowing what to expect from a small clinic in a town that was best known as a European resort.

Cherie was encouraged, though, and I could think of no good reason not to explore this. We'd been given the odds of traditional treatment on our home turf, and bottom line: those odds were not acceptable.

At this point, Trey had a surgery date scheduled several weeks out to remove his lung and follow up with IL-2 treatment in Atlanta. With the new possibility in Germany, we had to step up and quickly decide what to do. We knew his doctors here wouldn't be sending us off with any words of encouragement. While we were weighing things, Coach Hepler and leaders from Browns Bridge Community Church pulled together a prayer meeting. It met on the football field of West Forsyth's stadium. To our gratitude, it drew numerous friends, teammates, and community members who came together to pray for us as we struggled to make a staggering decision. It was amazing; we were so overwhelmed by the support and concern. Standing in the middle of the football field, surrounded by all those people, it became very clear that going to Germany was the right decision. The possibility gave way to reality, and it was happening soon.

To some, I guess that removing Trey's lung seemed like a reasonable and fast way to rid him of melanoma, but I had my doubts. This disease was aggressive and my biggest question regarding lung removal was the same one my wife had. What if cancer came back in the other lung?

With that always a possibility, we wanted a non-surgical option that might prove to be more than a temporary fix, but wouldn't leave us with nothing to fall back on if it didn't work. I was upset that some people actually thought we were pursuing the non-surgical route because lung removal would end Trey's football days. Sports were the farthest thing from our minds when we considered our options. Football had nothing to do with the decision. Trey getting to play would only be a bonus if the treatment in Germany did what we hoped: enable his immune system to attack the cancer he already had and get rid of anything else that could be waiting to appear later.

Besides, football wasn't looking too promising at that point. If Trey got approved for the immunepheresis, he would be spending most of his senior year and football season in Germany. We hoped Trey would be able to stay on track to graduate with his classmates, though. These were the kids he had gone to school with since early elementary school days. We wanted what he wanted, which was to walk across the stage with them. Bob Carnaroli, head guidance counselor at West Forsyth, got very creative in designing a plan to help make Trey's graduation doable, provided that side effects from any treatments didn't leave Trey too sick to keep up.

I don't remember any family or friends trying to talk us out of going to Germany. Given the odds, and the likely outcome of staying put and moving forward with the IL-2 treatment plan, there didn't seem to be much of a choice. It was the only treatment plan that offered any real hope.

Cherie got on the phone with her dad. His encouragement was our final prompt to make plane reservations and decide on a place to stay. Those two actions really set the trip in motion. Because July is the beginning of high holiday season in Europe, I initially had a hard time finding us a place to stay, but it worked out and plans swiftly fell into place. Dr. Lentz was quick to respond to us and agreed to evaluate him immediately. Cherie's mother and sister came down from Kentucky and took the lead in caring for things on the home front, which included taking Wes back with them until we could figure out a long-term plan. Even though we were pretty much working on faith and belief that there were a lot of "God things" popping up around us, seeing the details pan out so fast was reassuring. It confirmed and validated that we were making the right decision for Trey.

Thankfully, our passports were up-to-date because of Cherie and the boys taking annual spring break cruises with other neighborhood moms and kids. Cherie's work was in a slow phase, and I had been laid off by my employer several months earlier due to the economy, so the timing was all the better.

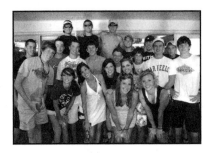 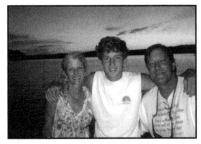

One last big summer blast with close friends before flying out to Germany (Trey in back row, wearing a hat and no shirt).

All that was left to do was cancel Trey's surgery. Regardless of either of our careers or jobs we did or didn't have at the time, we knew we had to find a way to make this work financially. All we could think of was doing whatever it took to help Trey survive. We had sold my NAPA Auto Parts business in Dawsonville several years earlier, and had put that money away in savings. This was the easiest money to use to make the trip to Germany happen. We were willing to give up anything and everything it took to fight for Trey's life, and figure out all the details later. The decision-making was very fast, because it had to be.

As we prepped to leave town, we honestly had no idea what we were doing. We just knew we had to do it. We left the country on July 11, 2009, two days after the prayer event at West Forsyth and three days before Trey would have had surgery before following up with IL-2 treatments.

Chapter Five

Trey

I was seventeen years old, and I just wanted to divide my summer between the football field and a wakeboard, so I pretty much hated Germany before our plane even landed. Even if I had been going for reasons other than cancer treatments, I probably would have been the unhappiest passenger on the whole transatlantic flight. I'm kind of a homebody anyway, and Germany was a long way from home. Still, with my doctors giving me a five percent chance for a cure and Germany upping the odds to fifty percent, I knew I needed to go.

I hoped my brother was going to be okay. He was going into his sophomore year at West Forsyth, a rising star in football and lacrosse. I had just assumed the summer days would kick off with me driving us to morning football workouts. I wondered, too, what this sudden change of plans was going to do to my chances of playing football in college. Once again, I just wished, more than anything, to be a normal teenager with normal concerns. It wasn't in the cards at that very moment, but I figured the sooner I got to Germany and underwent the treatment, the sooner I could get back to what felt right.

We knew before the trip that I was looking at a stay of two to four months, maybe even longer. It was possible my entire senior fall semester and football season would be spent on foreign turf, where I wasn't even sure Germans understood what American football was. The good news was that my treatment would be given on an outpatient basis. The bad news was that

I'd only get out after being hooked up to a machine for five to seven hours a day, five days a week. I planned to catch up on my sleep.

Even though I was walking around with the worst stage of melanoma, I still felt like I could step onto the football field and play. From what we were told by Dr. Lentz, the treatment wouldn't knock me flat from side effects. He said I'd probably feel like I had a touch of the flu while hooked up to the machine, and then fine once it was over with for the day.

That being the case, I was hoping I'd be allowed to make a quick trip home in late August for our season opener against cross-county rival North Forsyth Raiders. West Forsyth was still too new a school to say we were "longtime" rivals with North Forsyth, but we might as well have been. Most of us on the team had played against these guys while growing up, and that made the competition even fiercer. The urge to beat each other was as strong as two teams that had been facing each other down for fifty years. Actually, I guess I was more than hoping I'd be able to come home for that game; I was really counting on it.

Getting ready to leave for Germany was tense. It was like everything was happening in a video being shown at fast speed. My Aunt Ann (Mom's sister) was there to drive my parents and me to the airport. Once we got the luggage packed into the SUV, we headed down our familiar street. It was a quiet Saturday morning, at least until we got to a cross street not far from our house. Gathered on the corner was a cluster of about thirty people, holding up painted signs that read: We Love Trey, Praying for Trey, and Beten Sie fur Trey ("Praying for Trey" in German).

The crowd of friends, parents, and neighbors sent us off with so much support and love, I was humbled. Mom and I both jumped out of the SUV

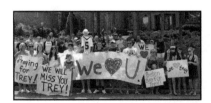 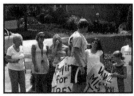 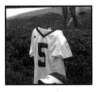

An amazing neighborhood sendoff to Germany!

and hurried into the crowd, where there were hugs and well-wishes. Dad, I think, was too choked up to move. He sat in the SUV and watched.

Cherie

Charlie and I knew our youngest son, Wes, had not gone untouched by Trey's illness. From day one, Wes's life had been rocked and altered along with the rest of ours, but he had always shown himself to be pretty strong. He and Trey were close, and Wes was hurting deeply. He didn't know how to help, and kept a lot of feelings locked up inside.

It was the morning we were rushing about, preparing to leave for Germany, when this wrenching realization, sharp as a knife, cut through my heart. Watching us get into the car was the point where Wes broke down, unable to hold his fears and pain back any longer. It hit him that we were really leaving, and it was more than he could handle. He sobbed, and as much as I wanted to cry with him, I knew I had to stay strong and focused on what we were doing: crossing an ocean to a foreign country and to a clinic I could only imagine.

I knew my mom and sister were going to be around to support Wes. He will be okay. We will all be okay. I kept telling myself that, believing we were doing the right thing. I had that gut feeling that God was leading us in the right direction, and would also take care of Wes.

Still, at the moment we were pulling out of the driveway, I saw (and knew) that Wes was not okay. With fear and confusion all over his face, he watched his mother, father, and only brother leave for an undetermined amount of time. I could only imagine how abandoned he must have felt. Worse, he couldn't completely understand any of this, or know what Trey might be like when he returned.

Seeing friends at the end of the street was a wonderful and encouraging send-off. Wes and my mother had walked down to be part of it, but Wes was not down on the street with the rest of the crowd. He stood up on the hill in the yard alongside my mother, looking terrified. Later she told me he asked if Trey was going to live. Watching his brother and his parents leave the country under a cloud of such urgency, he needed to know that we were all coming home to him.

With another son seriously ill, and a plane waiting to carry us over the ocean to a small clinic of hope, I could only cry seeing Wes break down. I felt so bad leaving him. I worried about the effect this would have on him. All I could do is look over the crowd.

"Someone take care of Wes!" I pleaded. My heart was breaking for him. My mother promised me she would. I could leave with that comfort, but I struggled with guilt and concern about not being there for him. I vowed we would send for him soon, that before school started he would join us in Germany for a visit. Though it wasn't the way I ever envisioned the four of us experiencing Europe together, the key word was together—we would be there as a family.

Wes

The day Mom, Dad, and Trey left for Germany was the worst one I'd had up to that point. First, everything with the trip happened so fast that I couldn't wrap my head around it. Suddenly, everyone was leaving—except me. It hit me that morning that I might not see them for a month or so. Saying goodbye was tough. At that point, nobody knew how things would come together. All that mattered was getting Trey to Germany as soon as possible.

I was all for them going, though. It seemed like the right thing to them, so it was the right thing to me. I still don't think I fully comprehended how sick Trey really was, though. He acted so normal when he was around me. Nothing about his outer appearance made him look sick. It was hard to believe there was anything wrong.

Right after we found out the melanoma was back, a guy at school walked up to me outside of the field house and said, "Hey Wes, man, I'm sorry Trey didn't get better news."

I must have really been hoping the news wasn't true, because I replied,

"Well, there's a chance they could have gotten his scans mixed up with somebody else's report. They could call and tell us that any day."

Of course, that call never came. Before I knew it, my family was leaving. Even though I still didn't know all the facts and details of Trey's melanoma, I did know it was more serious this time. The thing that had kept me most hopeful about Trey was Trey himself, but now I wouldn't be seeing and hearing from him every day. I guess it conjured up an image of life without him. For the first time, I wondered if this disease was something Trey might actually die from.

I was so glad to have Grandmom with me. Trey and I were very close to her, as well as to Neanie, my dad's mom. I felt even closer to them during the months they took turns staying with me. I also had my Aunt Ann, who helped me a lot. During the scariest times, when I texted her that I couldn't sleep, she would send me prayers.

I know Mom and Dad worried about me, and how I'd be affected by them not being around. It was hard, but I knew they wished they didn't have to be away. They had to be with Trey. If it had been me who was sick instead, I know they would have been with me just as much. My family was given a terrible ordeal, but I knew I was left in the best care.

Grandmom Barbara Arnold Simms

When my grandson asked me, "Is Trey going to die?" I wanted to give him one hundred percent assurance that Trey would come home completely healed. We all wished for that assurance, but we would have to wait and see. I told Wes the truth was that Trey had a terrible disease and would undergo many treatments.

"We're going to church to pray about it," I told him.

I understood my daughter's stance on keeping everything positive. The mind can go to the worst places. It can spiral, going down so fast that you can't catch it. Prayer can stop the spiral from starting, and that was very important for Wes. The breakdown in the woods was proof that he was hurting and had been keeping a lot of feelings inside. He and Trey are very close, but in the quest to get Trey well, Wes was the one getting left behind. I knew he felt helpless, so I tried to build him up and remind him of how many people loved him.

The news that Trey had cancer affected me on two levels. I hurt for my own child, Cherie, as well as for my grandson. When the cancer returned as stage IV, I traveled from my home in Louisville to be with them in Georgia. I was there when they made the decision to go to Germany. We were all hopeful, but knew it could be a long, difficult road for the family. It took all of us helping each other to get through it.

At one point during this time, I was having trouble sleeping, and feared a panic attack was coming on. The timing was interesting, because I was writing a devotional for my missionary circle at church, and the topic was peace. I prayed a lot about my lack of peace. The person who used to help me was one of the people I was worrying so much about—Trey. He reminded me of the Bible scriptures that tell us not to worry, and why. After that, I was able to say what Trey always said about his own set of circumstances: "I'm going to be all right."

Trey was such a faithful, mature, and non-complaining seventeen-year-old who also told me that he was "willing to accept what God does." I would say, "Trey, I'm so anxious to see how the Lord will use you."

Cherie

Charlie and I found Prien am Chiemsee, Germany, to be both quaint and bold, a village of shops and restaurants that are authentically Bavarian, and a place of resounding church bells and Old World flower boxes gracing windows. It's set against a scenic view of the majestic Upper Bavarian Alps that calls both tourists and locals to hike and bike its passes. The village languishes on the western shore of the deep blue Chiemsee Lake, which is also called the Bavarian Sea even though it's freshwater. I don't think the many people who were sailing, swimming, skiing, and enjoying every other kind of watery recreation were too concerned about that, though. They all seemed to be making the most of their vacations. We, on the other hand, arrived armed and ready with our English-to-German translation book. We tried to follow the instructions of the German-speaking navigation system in our extra-small diesel car, a two-door stick shift that displayed everything in kilometers. Charlie is a backseat driver and a wealth of what I call "useless trivia," but it does come in handy at times. Pulling from what he had learned from a television special about how to drive on the autobahn (Germany's freeway system) he would tell me what speeds to reach and maintain, though cars were still whizzing by and leaving us in the dust. When you are having a hard time believing you're actually in Germany, finding yourself on the autobahn will certainly snap you back into reality.

Our hotel room in Prien pretty much redefined the term "close quarters": four hundred square feet housing a king-size bed, a twin, and a pullout sofa. It also had a separate room that rivaled the size of a closet, which Trey chose as his space. It did have two windows, though, that overlooked the village maypole and the main church, and offered a stunning view of the Alps. The room's only amenity was a tiny refrigerator that was just big enough to squeeze in Trey's Cokes and Charlie's beer.

Of course, our first major stop, and focal point of our stay, was the small Lentz Praxis clinic, where Dr. Lentz, his wife Dr. Kiran Lentz, and their colleagues were devoted to immunepheresis. (It was called "Lentz Praxis" in German, but in English it essentially meant "Lentz practice clinic.") The doctors worked with patients from all over the world with various types of cancers, most of them in stage IV. Yet, despite the many patients who had entered its doors before us, Trey may have been the youngest to ever turn to them for help.

Trey

My new hospital was nothing like the ones I was used to at home. Lentz Praxis was so small that Dr. Lentz gave us the tour himself. I really liked him. He was optimistic and said he could push me hard because I was young. Thanks to football, I wasn't afraid of hard work. He was also encouraged that

I had never been through chemo or radiation, since those aren't ordinary treatments for my type of cancer. My body wasn't torn down and exhausted by them. Dr. Lentz also wasn't used to seeing patients with my body type. At first, he was concerned when a CT scan showed what looked like a thick area around my liver that was pressing against my stomach. The radiologist confirmed it was muscle tissue, better known as a "six-pack." They also said my pulse was healthier than what they were used to seeing, and the nurses nicknamed it my "sports pulse."

Other great news that came early on was that the CT scan showed the tumor in my lung hadn't grown since the PET scan in mid-June, and no new tumors had shown up. Dr. Lentz was really upbeat about having me there. I don't think he saw me as a guinea pig or anything, but he definitely seemed to think I was a good candidate for immunepheresis. I got the feeling he was putting all effort into a successful treatment. All the way around, I was very hopeful I'd walk out of there just the way Mom kept telling me I would: cancer-free, with no surgery or ICU time back in Atlanta. That's not to say my attitude about being in Germany was getting any better, though. I still didn't like it. Being away from my family and friends back home was very hard.

I was the only kid of all the patients seen that summer. The closet person to my age was still more than twenty years older than me, and everyone else was in their fifties and sixties. We all had one big thing in common, though:

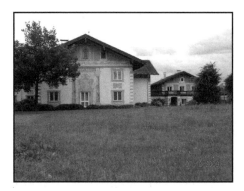

The Lentz-Praxis Clinic (Prien am Chiemsee, Germany).

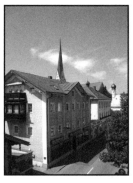

View from Rood family hotel room in Prien am Chiemsee, Germany.

being in stage IV of some type of cancer. My fellow patients were Americans from all over the United States, and most had family members or friends who had come to Germany with them. Everyone was friendly and helpful, and Mom quickly realized that they would be our German family. She spent a lot of time hanging out with them in the family room at the clinic, because Dr. Lentz didn't allow any visitors to sit in the treatment area with patients. If you knew my mom, you'd know she wasn't happy about that. The doctor didn't bend the rules for me, even though I was considered a minor. Mom and Dad were only allowed to occasionally walk back to the doorway and look in on me for a minute or two.

I wasn't crazy about the treatment area, either. Maybe that was because I'd been spoiled by the big facilities in Atlanta. Lentz Praxis was like a small sardine can in comparison, with only three patient treatment rooms for those undergoing immunepheresis. Each room had three beds, and on a lot of days, three patients in each room sharing the cramped space. Of course, given the shoebox space that I had back at the hotel, maybe a room that could hold three people was spacious and sprawling by European standards.

Dr. Lentz told me to plan on being at the clinic every weekday for the first three weeks from nine to five, hooked up to the immunepheresis machine with breaks every ninety minutes or so. "Boring" was the word that came to mind when I learned of my daily routine. I'm pretty sure that's the first word that comes to anyone's mind, so I don't think my age had anything to do with how little I looked forward to the treatment.

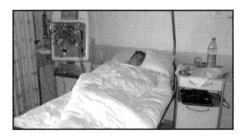

Long days of treatment at Lentz-Praxis.

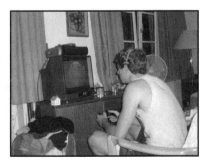

Long nights of play on the Xbox in Trey's hotel room.

I quickly decided that I would sleep through the long days by staying up all night playing Xbox and Facebooking with my friends at home. Germany was six hours ahead of the Atlanta time zone, so that was actually perfect timing. I could talk to Wes and my teammates and coaches about how football workouts and practices were going. Once the two-a-day practices started, I could sign on around three in the morning my time, and talk to the guys shortly after they got home around nine that night their time. I figured that would help me feel more connected to the team, like I was still in the loop.

Mom and Dad took what was probably a life-threatening drive on the autobahn to find a store where they could buy a European Xbox for me. It had to plug into a German outlet to work. They only blew one fuse at the hotel, but Mom said it got me to smile and that was worth a million bucks to them. While it wasn't easy being seventeen and stuck some place I didn't want to be, I'm sure it also wasn't easy being around me, either.

Chapter Six

Charlie

Trey's spirits were pretty down the first week in Germany, to the point that Dr. Lentz expressed his concerns to Cherie and me. The Xbox actually proved to be medicinal for that, though, because it lets kids play games against each other wherever they happen to be in the world. Being online with his brother and buddies seemed to be what Trey wanted to do most with his time in Germany.

We found the Xbox at a store in Rosenheim, Germany, which is a city about thirty minutes away from Prien am Chiemsee, and is the seat of administration for the Upper Bavaria region. It was also rumored that a poltergeist haunted it in the late 1960s. Investigations never proved whether the alleged paranormal activity was faked. Cherie and I didn't see anything that struck us as being paranormal, but we saw plenty in Germany that seemed abnormal—like beer sold in hospital vending machines, and nice restaurants where it was insulting to waiters if you tipped them more than five percent! I still haven't figured that one out. There were plenty of shops, and Cherie quickly figured out that "SALE" is spelled the same way in Germany as it is back home.

The very first step at the clinic was to have a catheter line placement implanted into Trey's chest so that his blood could be withdrawn, then filtered through the immunepheresis machine and returned—similar to standard dialysis treatments. Trey's early side effects from the immunepheresis were pretty much contained to a low-grade fever. On the fourth day, though, he came down with a case of the shakes in addition to the fever. Dr. Lentz told us this was a good indicator the treatment was working, forcing Trey's immune system to go into overdrive. It was too soon to tell if it was fighting against the cancer, but we were reassured that his body reacting to treatment was a positive sign.

Overall, we found the medical world to be a lot more relaxed in Germany than it is in the United States. Right after Trey woke up from surgery, we took him to the hospital down the street for a CT scan, where he alternated drinking contrast solution and Coca-Cola just before the test. Cherie was even allowed to sit with the CT technician and watch the computer screen while pictures and data were being gathered.

Unfortunately, the cost of being in Germany was higher than you can imagine, and not just the twenty euros (about thirty United States dollars) it took for the three of us to eat dinner at the nearest McDonalds. The immunepheresis cost eighty thousand dollars per month—cash only—and we had no help at all from our insurance carrier since it was an alternative treatment, conducted outside the United States. Back home, friends and family were working to raise whatever funds they could to take some of the burden off, starting with a pancake breakfast and silent auction sponsored by the West Forsyth football boosters. Those must have been some good pancakes, because the club raised thirty-eight thousand dollars to be used as needed for Trey. We were very grateful for every dime and the relief it gave us.

Despite a tight budget, we tried to make the best of our time over there. When Trey was off the immunepheresis machine, he felt pretty good, which meant his weekends had potential for being enjoyable. Most of the clinic's

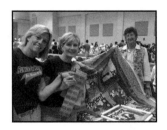

Trey's Grandmom, Jean Jones (standing, right), made this quilt to sell at a silent-auction fundraiser.

patients and their families tried to get out and explore the area, which is exactly what Cherie and I wanted to do. Trey's sense of adventure didn't quite match ours, though. He showed little interest in anything that kept him from the Xbox or computer, his connections to life back home.

Cherie

Charlie and I did insist that Trey get out some during our first weekend in Germany. Saturday was gloomy and gray, with a steady rain that seemed to shrink our hotel room ever smaller, if that was possible. It was a good day for resting, though, so we let Trey have Saturday by doing something most teenagers are very good at—sleeping. Sunday was cool and overcast, so we decided to venture up to the Kehlsteinhaus (more commonly known in America as the "Eagle's Nest"), a historic chalet-style mountain retreat still standing from the days of Hitler and the Third Reich. There's no question how it got its name, perched high on a peak in the Bavarian Alps on the border of Germany and Austria. We had heard the panoramic views of the mountain range were unbelievably stunning.

Trey wasn't as enthused about this day trip as Charlie and I, and didn't expect to be overly impressed by the view that awaited us. Still, he was a good sport and came along without complaining, for which I was grateful. From the moment we arrived in Germany, I trusted that faith had brought us there. It felt right. I was hopeful that Trey's cancer was going to be cured, and to protect that hope, I had built a wall around me that tolerated zero negativity.

Comic relief is always welcome during challenging times. I'm not sure you can survive without it, and our first legitimate German outing was ready to provide plenty of punch lines. It actually wasn't an outing as much as a wild goose chase. Our German-speaking navigation system turned a planned one-hour drive into two-and-a-half hours of zigzagging on skinny mountain roads in and out of two countries. We crossed over into Austria twice. The second time, our tiny car got hit by a horse.

Coming around the narrow bend of a curvy road, we faced off with two people riding horseback. An equine head-on collision looked unavoidable.

Though one of those horses alone could have probably stepped on and squashed our tiny car, both animals freaked out at the sight of us. We managed to stop, but the riders couldn't bring one horse under control before he ran right into the car. Thankfully, no harm was done to the animal or our tin can.

When we finally made it to the Eagle's Nest, we were greeted by granite walls, heavy wooden ceiling beams, and a grand interior. We saw the room where Eva Braun, Hitler's longtime companion, entertained, as well as the red marble fireplace that Mussolini gave to Hitler. The most fascinating thing waited thousands of feet above us and was only accessible by a twenty-minute bus ride (or a grueling two-and-a half-hour hike). We boarded the bus and crept along a steep road that took us 2,275 feet into the sky before dropping us off at a the entrance of a long, cold, marble-lined tunnel that led through Kehlstein Mountain. A the end of the tunnel was a mirrored elevator that swiftly shot us airborne another four hundred feet before opening its doors to reveal that we still had another three hundred feet to go.

We had to walk that last bit, but emerged on the summit for the promised three-hundred-and-sixty-degree view of the jagged and towering Alps, breathtaking in their blue hues and snow caps—the powerful sculpting and craftsmanship of God's fingers. As predicted, Trey wasn't moved by the sight quite the way Charlie and I were, but we believe it was a moment he would remember forever. We took in the view from every angle and admired all facets of it, but had to laugh when we suddenly felt like the Griswalds in

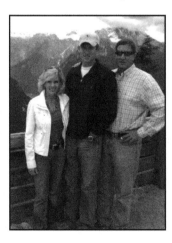

Cherie, Trey, and Charlie take a weekend excursion between treatments to see the Eagle's Nest, Hitler's hideaway.

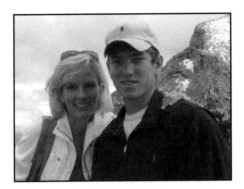

Cherie and Trey pose on excursion to Eagle's Nest in Germany.

European Vacation. After all the time and effort it took to reach the summit, and after seeing what there was to see, we wrapped it up with: "Well, we've been here and done this. Now it's time to leave.

Down the mountain we went, and back into the car we crawled, to wind our way back down to our temporary home in Prien am Chiemsee. Poor Trey got sick from all the twists and turns in the road, and we pulled over briefly to let him out. Next, we had to look for a gas station that would take a credit card, which is not always easy to find in a land that favors cash-only transactions. We were counting out our last ten euros due to some unexpected medical expenses. Fortunately, there was a credit-friendly gas station along the way, so we didn't get stranded on the side of the road. Thankfully, too, Wes was on his way from the United States, which worked out much sooner than we thought we'd be able to have him visit. Luckily, my dad had found a way to transfer money to Dodi Mace, a close friend and neighbor who was flying with Wes. She literally carried the cash on the plane.

Wes's impending arrival was such a bright spot, as was the fact that he was traveling with Dodi and her daughter Cailin. We couldn't wait to see this lively trio arrive later the next day, and the anticipation made our dinner at the hotel that night even more enjoyable.

With our first week in Germany behind us, we geared up for Trey's second week of treatment, scheduled to begin the next morning. Before bed, I administered a shot that would elevate his white blood cell count, the prick of the needle a reminder of where we really were.

Chapter Seven

Cherie

Trey's second week in Germany began with the not-so-welcome news that he needed to switch to a sugar-free diet to promote a healthy immune system. Like most mothers, I've often told my boys they need to eat right, but finding something sugar-free that passes a teenager's taste test never comes without challenges.

Goodie boxes from family and friends back home had already begun to arrive, and were filled with all the sweet treats a teenager could love. In fact, we had just opened one packed with candy, Oreo cookies, Pop Tarts and other confections. Then Dr. Kiran Lentz (Dr. Lentz's wife and coordinator of the treatment's nutrition program) sat me down to talk about Trey's dietary needs. She had already prescribed him a variety of daily vitamins, but said it was time to take all sugar off the menu. As far as sweets go, only dark chocolate was on the approved list. It quickly became the treat Trey looked forward to every day. He was also allowed nuts and organic fruits that were, thankfully, easy to find in the local grocery stores.

Trey accepted the dietary changes just as he had accepted everything else related to his fight against cancer: not thrilled, but willing to do what was asked of him. The hardest thing for Trey to part with was the glass-bottled Cokes he could buy from the German vending machines. He loved them, claiming they tasted better than the Cokes in plastic and aluminum he was used to at home. Though he made the switch to sugar-free drinks, I knew he viewed it as a temporary condition. "Mom, when I get back home, I'll be eating anything I want to again," he informed me. "I'll be cancer-free."

In his mind, diet wouldn't matter once the cancer was gone. I had to love the resilient, fearless attitude of youth, but I knew we had some work to do in convincing him that the sugar-free diet needed to be a lifelong change. For the time being, though, I decided to focus on where we were in the present and take his sugarless lifestyle one day at a time. Though the contents of our care packages changed, they continued showing up every few days. People from my employer's home office mailed a box every week filled with snacks, magazines, and as many other comforts from home as they could pack inside. These wonderful gestures were like warm hugs from across the ocean and really brought a sense of peace, a reminder that we were loved and being thought of.

Using contents from one of the home packages, the first thing I cooked for Trey was some whole-wheat pasta with sugar-free tomato sauce. With no kitchen in our hotel room, I boiled the pasta at the clinic, towed it back to the hotel, and had the hotel staff warm it up with the sauce. Boy, you sure do learn to never take the comforts of home for granted again! Trey ate every bite of the ultra-healthy dish without putting up a fight or even making faces to express his sugarless disgust. That was progress, and once again, reminded me that we could do this.

Trey's spirits lifted somewhat that second week. The arrival of Wes, Dodi, and Cailin was a highlight, and they came bearing gifts to make Trey's "nanosuite" more homey. University of Georgia (UGA) linens and decorations converted the bland quarters into a haven of red and black. Dodi and the kids added West Forsyth touches, like Trey's team picture and a blanket. Dodi also negotiated a different refrigerator to replace the small one in our room. Catching sight of a hotel employee moving a regular-size one into the building, she somehow got it redirected to our room, making it much easier to keep drinks cold and store some of Trey's medications.

While the new families we met were incredible, and they understood our journey on a deep level because of similar paths, it was therapeutic to see familiar faces from home. Dodi was quick to take care of tasks that, at times, seemed overwhelming to me, like scooping up our dirty laundry and hauling it out for cleaning. She put together a small birthday celebration for

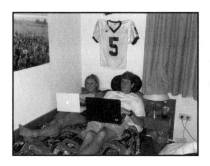

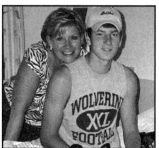

Childhood friend Cailin Mace and Trey "connecting" from their respective laptops in the hotel.

Dodi Mace and Trey in Prien am Chiemsee, Germany.

Charlie, making it festive with a cake, decorations, and lots of laughter when we discovered that the German print on the balloons she bought actually read "Cordial on Your Wedding Day!" instead of "Happy Birthday!"

Dodi also walked me over to the Catholic church across the street from our hotel, where we admired the magnificent frescos, ornate trim work, and (more than anything else) the air conditioning. Other than a bank Charlie and I had stopped by, this was the only place in town we found to offer cool refuge against the summer heat. Dodi and I approached the altar, said prayers for Trey, sprinkled ourselves with holy water, and stood in quiet awe of our surroundings.

Trey was happy to have the company of his brother and good friend. Hearing them laugh, piled in Trey's tiny room, was music to my ears and reminded me of life back home. It was a glimpse of the pre-cancer years. It was also a glimpse into what I firmly expected to be a cancer-free future. Because of his treatments, Trey wasn't able to join them on any sightseeing trips. He did enjoy their evenings together playing old-fashioned American board games, like Scattergories, and working on a complicated, thousand-piece puzzle a family we met at the clinic gave us.

By day ten of his treatment, Trey was consistently feeling the expected side effects of chills and shakes, high fevers, headaches, and soreness in the area of his left lung where the tumor was. Again, we were told this was an encouraging sign that the treatment was working on his system. The first round of treatment would officially end once he moved through day fourteen. At that point, he'd get a break for a few days, then a CT scan to check his progress. If all went well, the scan would show less tumor in his left lung and he would enter the second round of treatment: another twelve days like the first round.

Trey

Right before I finished my first round of treatment, Wes and our friends had to go back to the United States. We had been in Germany just over two weeks. Dad, too, needed to make a brief trip home to take care of some matters and get Wes ready for his sophomore year, which began in early August. It was just Mom and me in Germany for a little while, though my Aunt Ann was coming over very soon. I can't describe how much I wanted to head to the airport with the others, but Mom tried really hard to make our "home away from home" as comfortable as possible. At this point, we didn't know just how long we would continue to stay in Germany—whether Dad would be flying back to us, or whether Mom and I would be coming home soon. We had to wait for the first round of CT scans after my first treatment was over to know if we would stay on for another three weeks to do a second round of immunepheresis. If the results came back showing some improvement in my right lung tumor or that things had stabilized, we would stay. Otherwise, there was no point in continuing treatment, so we'd return home.

We could only get one television station in English: CNN, for news and weather coverage. We watched some movies and DVDs of the *Friends* TV show, plus played some cards. Mom tried to make my diet change easier to take, too, and called it "huge progress" when I actually ate some almonds and raw carrots. She wanted me to eat salads with her, too, but they just seemed like useless food to me since they wouldn't help me keep my weight up.

Losing weight was a real concern to me because of football. Getting back to the game was a definite focus that helped me face the treatments I was going through. I was determined to get home for the game against North

Forsyth—and even hoped Dr. Lentz would clear me to play. For the time being, though, the football my Aunt Ann sent me was as close as I could get to the field. But it was cool, because another patient named Steven Shailer (who was forty-one and from Fort Lauderdale, Florida) invited me to go out behind the clinic and throw the ball around some. While that might not sound like a big deal to a lot of people, it was one of the best offers I'd had since arriving in Germany. We even had spectators. I guess the nurses weren't used to seeing patients play American football in their backyard. They were lined up at the window cheering. One of my favorite nurses, a guy named George, even ran to get his phone so he could take pictures.

Mom kept coming up with suggestions to get me out and active during the week off I had between first and second round treatments. Golf at a local course, hiking the Alps, and even trying out a nearby canopy zip line were some of her ideas, but what I was most interested in was weight training. I was missing all the summer football workouts at school—plus totally eliminating sugar from my diet was making it hard to keep weight on. Training and staying strong was a major priority, no matter what melanoma said, so Mom found a gym that would let us buy short-term memberships. I wanted her to go with me, figuring she'd like the treadmill while I used the weights.

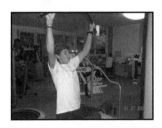

Trey working out at a local gym in Prien.

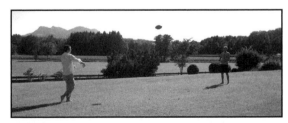

Steven Shailer, a fellow Lentz-Praxis patient, throws the ball with Trey out on the grass (Prien am Chiemsee, Germany).

Anything I could do to get me ready and back in time for football was worth it, and took a front seat to all other activities, which is why I didn't complain much about the treatment even though I hated it. As we headed into August, I was wrapping up round one and thinking about the kids at home who were getting ready to go back to school. It was hard to believe it was my senior year and I wouldn't be there with friends I'd been classmates with since my early elementary years.

It's weird, but *Why me?* never crossed my mind in the way some people might think. I did wonder why melanoma had chosen me, but it was more about what God wanted me to do with this experience. I absolutely felt called to something, and kind of knew that this was all happening for a reason.

I was sometimes curious about what my friends really thought of all of this. They were always supportive, but one of the ways they supported me was by acting normal whenever they came around. That was what I wanted, and I appreciated it. They wouldn't bring up cancer unless I did. Since I hardly ever did, it wasn't something that got discussed very much. Cailin was one of my closest friends from way back, but I was also tight with two guys named Nathan Teter and Joey Moran. This had to have impacted them. It's not every day a good friend you've grown up with gets cancer while you're all still kids.

Joey Moran

I met Trey right after he moved into our neighborhood, back in second grade. We were on the same Midway Park Packers football team for the seven-to-eight-year-old group. Pretty soon, we were playing baseball together on the Forsyth Diamondbacks and Midway Vipers teams. We grew very close during those years. My mother and Mrs. Cherie shared carpool duties to get us to all of our games in various places.

When our community first heard that Trey had cancer, everyone was in shock. I remember how concerned all the parents in the neighborhood were, how involved everyone became, and how fast plans to help came together and took place. Being so young, though, I didn't quite understand how life-threatening Trey's stage of melanoma actually was. When he was diagnosed with stage IV later in high school, I had a better idea by then, and it was heartbreaking.

Trey was one of the best athletes West Forsyth had seen to this point. He was also the epitome of humble and down-to-earth. Most importantly to me, Trey turned into one of the most inspiring people in my life. He never got down on himself, despite the hand he was dealt. No matter where he might have stood mentally while getting treatment, he stayed positive and had a great outlook on life.

Trey might have been hurting physically during parts of his treatment, but you would have never guessed that just from looking at him. He was so mentally strong and so set on overcoming this challenge that no obstacle in his path was going to stop him from being rid of cancer. He believed he needed to overcome these obstacles to prove a point to people: No matter how bad the circumstances might be, never give up faith in the Lord. Keep the faith and He will guide you through whatever it is.

Besides faith, I believe the main reason behind Trey's relentless effort to fight cancer was the love and care from his family and his friends. The overall outlook of the people we went to school with was relatively positive. The majority who knew Trey believed that he would overcome melanoma and get back to being the athlete he used to be. I know that the people closest to Trey naturally worried more than anyone else. When Trey went to Germany, Cailin and I constantly said prayers for him and Skyped with him whenever we could. It was always good, and reassuring, to see him and know that he was okay. I also played Xbox games online with him while he was overseas—anything to make him feel more comfortable and normal.

Trey really hated missing football practice that summer. A lot of guys were always looking for a day off, but Trey would have given anything to be out there on the field, even in the miserable heat. Football is one of those sports that can serve to prepare an athlete for hard times, and I really saw it working in Trey. One of our old coaches used to preach the "Three Ds" mentality to us and it was very clear that it stuck with Trey. "You gotta have the Three D's," the coach would say. "Dedication, determination, and the desire to achieve whatever hand you're dealt." Trey exemplified this during his illness.

It was important to Trey that he just be a regular guy like the rest of us. The last thing he wanted was special treatment, or worse, any kind of pity. I learned that the best thing I could do for him was to avoid bringing up cancer whenever we were together. All of his good friends felt that way, so unless he started talking about his treatment or situation, none of us did. We'd just act like nothing was different and it was a normal day. Nobody had to fake it or work at being normal, though. Trey was still Trey: steady, someone you could just easily hang out and talk with. His attitude didn't change or bounce around to extremes, no matter what doctors and medical reports said. He had faith that he would overcome this cancer, and that was his focus.

Nathan Teter

I also met Trey when he moved into the neighborhood around second grade. We were on the same school bus, and had a lot in common as far as our personalities and interest in sports. The real connection between Trey and me, though, started out on the football field when we were eight years old. That's when we became close friends. We were soon inseparable. We continued to play on the same football team throughout high school.

When I first found out Trey had been diagnosed with melanoma, I was more in shock than anything. First, I didn't know much at all about melanoma and how serious it was. Also, I had never had a relative or friend, at that point, have their life put in jeopardy. Everyone around me stayed so positive about Trey, though, that I just told myself he would be cured and things would get back to normal again. It was when the melanoma returned as stage IV that it truly hit me that this was real. I broke down, not knowing where to turn. I just felt miserable, and couldn't fathom losing my best friend in high school.

I never saw Trey become negative about anything having to do with his situation. He always stayed so upbeat and optimistic about everything going on, which in turn made me feel optimistic about everything.

I believe the support Trey had behind him, coming from his faith, family, friends, and the community, as well as from football, kept him extremely motivated to keep on fighting. How someone can go through miserable cancer treatments and still perform at the level he did in football is beyond me.

In my eyes, the attitude from everyone around Trey was very positive.

Everyone just kind of doubted the statistics and believed he would pull through. Obviously, the odds that doctors originally gave Trey of surviving through high school worried many people. Yet, because of Trey's positive attitude and his will to keep fighting, he motivated others around him to stay positive and keep the faith.

I think a lot of what kept Trey motivated during treatment was the escape football gave him. For two hours a day, he felt disease-free and like any other one of our brothers on the field. The coaches were great in handling what was going on and always kept him, as well as the team, positive on all levels.

I also think football itself was a huge part of Trey's success in his battle with cancer. Not only did football keep Trey's physical health in peak condition for treatments, it also taught him how to fight through tough situations, to "embrace the grind." He didn't ask for this to happen to him, but he accepted it, believing he would overcome the odds and battle through it. Football teaches you to persevere through whatever is thrown your way, to fight to the last second of any tough situation. Trey has always had that attitude in everything he has done.

To me and others close to Trey, he was a normal teenager. Nobody changed the way they interacted with him. He was my best friend, we were still going to do everything we wanted to do, and cancer wasn't going to stop that. Of course, we talked about his treatments and progress, but we were normal teenagers having the time of our lives. Nothing changed about Trey's personality through his fight. He was still the same fun-loving guy he had always been.

One memory I'll have for the rest of my life is the day Trey got back from Germany after intense experimental treatment. I was at football practice and was so on edge about Trey's status from the treatments that I just wasn't feeling myself. I remember stretching on the field before practice, and seeing him walk down the stadium steps onto the football field. I had goose bumps for about ten minutes, I was so overjoyed to see my best friend was okay. At that moment, I knew Trey would make it through his battle and never questioned it again.

Charlie

Trying to fly back to the states during Europe's high holiday season can be looked at in two different ways: an adventure, or something to do only if you really need to get to America.

Dodi's husband Steve is a pilot with Delta Airlines, with more than twenty years of seniority. He made arrangements for Wes and me to use Buddy Passes to fly, which was a much-appreciated gesture. The only drawback was that we had to fly standby. We were traveling with Dodi and Cailin, and arrived at the Munich airport to find a complete madhouse. I was doubtful the four of us would be able to fly together, and the hordes of tourists meant we were in for a lot of standing on standby.

Two days passed, and we were still waiting to get on a plane. Deciding that a Munich-to-Atlanta flight might not happen until every last tourist in Europe was long gone, we boarded a train to Brussels, hoping for a better shot at that airport. The train ride took eight hours. We arrived in Brussels to find a similar packed situation, but about half the number of people we'd seen in the Munich airport.

Finally, some seats opened up, but only three. I sent Dodi, Cailin, and Wes on their way, and tried to find a flight for myself. At that point, I was willing to take a flight to anywhere in the United States. The smallest airport in the most remote corner of the country would have been fine with me. I knew once I landed somewhere in the states, making my way to Atlanta would be pretty easy, even if it meant renting a car and driving. I got out later in the day on a flight bound for New York City. Maybe as a little reward for all the stress, I actually ended up in business class, though I would have happily taken a lawn chair on the wing!

One of the toughest things about our new international lifestyle was deciding where to be and when. Cherie wasn't quite ready for me to leave her to deal with Germany on her own, but things at home were demanding attention. Mainly, there was Wes to consider. We would soon be transitioning between Cherie's mother returning to Kentucky and my mom arriving from North Carolina to keep an eye on him and the house. During his week with us in Germany, Wesley had worked on me some to return home with him for a little while. He'd been nothing but supportive and a good sport since the day Trey was first diagnosed a couple of years earlier, but Wes was only fifteen, and we knew he needed our time and attention as well. We decided I'd stay in town until his sophomore year got off to a start. Plus, I'd catch some of his football practices instead of just hearing about them.

I wanted to make the trip home for some much-needed one-on-one time with Wes, but was torn about leaving Trey before we even knew if the treatment was yielding any success. Cherie believed the clinic was where we were meant to be. We both liked the optimism of Dr. Lentz and the support of other American families. The patients at this clinic, though, had cancer cases that were among the worst of the worst, and this was their last option. It's tough to swallow that your child is sick enough to fall into the same category. He was also a new demographic to the clinic, so they had no cases to compare him to in that respect. I had to believe it was working, though, and our first indication came on August 7.

Chapter Eight

Cherie

The first week of August marked a welcome break from treatment, giving Trey some physical and mental relief from the long days he had been spending at the clinic. There was also a nervous energy in the air as we waited for the August 7 testing that would tell us if this trip to Germany was paying off.

My sister Ann arrived from the states for what we hoped would be a low-key visit. Unfortunately, she stepped off the plane to receive the message about my nephew Chris's watercraft accident. T-boned by another watercraft on a lake, he was in a Lima, Ohio hospital. This was a tough dilemma for Ann as she wrestled with staying in Germany with Trey and me, or catching the next flight to be with Chris.

She spent her first night in Germany on the phone, talking to doctors, and getting the assurance from family and friends that they were by her son's side. In the end, she decided to stay in Germany until August 10 as planned, meaning she would be with Trey and me when we got the good (or bad) results of his tests. While I would have certainly understood if Ann had turned around and gone back home, I was so appreciative that she chose to stay with us.

While the time in Germany was never about enjoying tourism, I tried to make the most out of our extended stay there. This was partly to ward off going stir-crazy in our tiny hotel room, but it also fit in with my goal to keep spirits lifted and attitudes positive. Between Trey's impending tests and Chris's accident, Ann and I both needed distractions to keep us sane.

The week was full of some interesting, if not strange, sights as I took Ann around to nearby villages. An elderly man riding his bike along a country road, dressed in nothing but loose-fitting tighty-whitey underwear, was one sight we probably could have gone our whole lives without seeing! The most shocking sight, though, was watching a two-year-old boy sip beer through his baby bottle. His parents later converted the bottle into a sippy cup by removing the lid and giving him a straw to drink his beer through. While this would have had Child Services swooping down hard in America, it didn't seem to raise eyebrows in Germany, other than mine and Ann's.

We also paid a visit to the English Garden (Englischer Garten) in Munich, which is the oldest and largest park in all of Europe. Size-wise, it's comparable to New York City's Central Park. We walked for what seemed like miles and miles. The sights included more than a few European sunbathers (mostly older men), sprawled out in the nude. Most people kept their clothes on, though, and we saw hundreds of them enjoying lively Bavarian music while sampling authentic German foods. The most fascinating attractions were the surfers, who took their colorful boards out on a river flowing through the park. I had never seen river surfing before, but strong rapids made the water perfect to show off their talents.

Trey wasn't too interested in going out with us, but we did convince him to join us for a gondola ride up a mountainside that came with a breathtaking view of the Bavaria region. While we were standing at the very top of the mountain, a massive storm suddenly churned up and spewed out what American meteorologists like to call "golf ball-size hail." It resembled big balls of popcorn bouncing about the mountain fields. The sight impressed Trey enough for him to call it "cool." We were glad that something about Germany had finally impressed him!

We also convinced Trey to join us for the popular German pastime of bike riding, which we did one afternoon in Prien. The countryside is filled with scenic bike trails weaving through the hills, meadow, and wooded areas. Though Trey didn't seem to want to admit that the trails were pretty awesome, he did ride along with no complaints. He also went with us to the large Catholic church across the street, where we prayed with him.

Finally, with no coaxing at all, he was treated to a night of five-star dining at the Residenz Heinz Winkler, an exquisite restaurant tucked amid Bavarian fairytale scenery between Salzburg and Munich. Heinz Winkler is the most-celebrated top chef in Germany, and his restaurant has been awarded three Michelin stars multiple times for its superb cuisine. This amazing dinner was compliments of Ann's Texas friend (now husband), Monte Bond, who wanted to reward Trey for hanging so tough during his treatments. Given the cost of those treatments, and the budget they required us to survive on, this night of fine dining was a real treat.

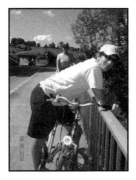

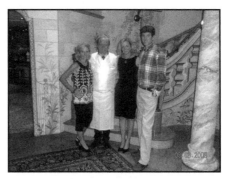

Trey stops to take a break in Germany during a bike riding excursion.

Cherie, Ann, and Trey pose with Grand Chef Heinz Winkler (Aschau im Chiemgau, Germany).

One of the best things to happen that week was Trey making a Skype call with friends back home. Kevin Ragsdale at Browns Bridge Community Church pulled off an incredible feat by putting Trey on Skype during the youth Bible worship service, called InSide Out, which allowed Trey to watch as well as interact. He was so excited to go to church via technology! He loved the service and praise music, and was truly uplifted by his friends. Kevin, who had been Trey's small-group leader for a couple of years, had absolutely proven to be a loyal friend and Christian mentor, one who Trey leaned on heavily for support and influence in his walk of faith. Kevin's idea to link Trey up with his friends was great medicine. I quickly realized that there wasn't a pastime or attraction in all of Europe that could have pulled more smiles and laughter from Trey than that hour or so "at church" did. Seeing the positive impact this had on him, I hoped it would become a weekly event for as long as we were in Germany.

Trey

Being Skyped into the high school services at church was cool. Kevin Ragsdale asked me to talk to the other kids about what I was going through, keeping it along the lines of "when bad things happen to good people." Even though there had been times during my illness when I didn't want to acknowledge anything connected to life with cancer, I really wanted to talk about my experience this time. This might have been when I started thinking my fight with melanoma had happened for a reason, and that maybe I was called to use it for some kind of good. Maybe God would heal me through these treatments in Germany, and that would give hope to others who were sick. On the other hand, maybe people who weren't sick would be inspired and extra-motivated to do things by watching a guy with stage IV melanoma manage to keep playing football and try to live like a normal teenager.

Many of the kids I spoke to that evening were ones I had known for a long time. I'd been part of the youth programs at Browns Bridge since middle school. I had gone to all of the retreats, and on a summer trip to Panama City, Florida, where leaders tried to get us fired up about God through praise services and speakers focused on topics pertinent to our age group—things like standing up to peer pressure, making good decisions, and putting God first in our lives.

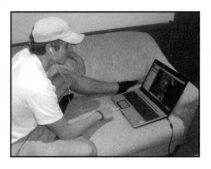

Trey Skyping with Brown's Bridge Community Church during their high school "InsideOut" worship service.

The last one—putting God first—was something I didn't do when I first started going to Browns Bridge. I believed in Him, but really didn't think about Him a whole lot in my everyday living. Even during my first fight, when the melanoma was in stage III, God didn't have my whole heart. That would change in a big way as I got into the fight with stage IV and began to understand that God had some kind of plan for everyone. He had one for me. Though I wasn't really sure what it was, I knew I was going to have to accept it and go with it. That's what I talked to the kids about that first night on Skype.

Nothing about the plan was going to make me love Germany, but I was happy on August 7 when the CT scan showed that I was making some progress. The tumor in my left lung was still the same size, but it was starting to show what Dr. Lentz called "liquefaction," which meant it might be dying in the center. I knew I still had a long way to go, but any progress was good, especially since I'd only been in treatment for a few weeks. I started the twelve-day session of round two of treatment. This time Mom and I ran to the clinic some days. It was only about two miles from our hotel, and I actually did a sprint-walk-sprint routine because it was just one more way to stay in shape for football.

This had suddenly become more important than ever, because Dr. Lentz decided I could go home for a couple of weeks after my second round was finished. I'd be getting back to Atlanta on August 27, just in time for the game against North Forsyth. It's hard to imagine how disappointed I would have been if Dr. Lentz had nixed that hope. Instead, I was ecstatic.

In her email update to our friends on August 11, Mom wrote: "No question God is working through Trey and our prayers are starting to be answered!!"

I was really believing it too.

Cherie

I wrote that email with complete faith that good things were happening for Trey. We even had possible medical evidence to back it up. Though the tumor's appearance of liquefaction was only a small glimmer of progress, we took it.

As Trey got a little further into round two of treatment, the cough he developed during the first round started to get slightly worse. His throat was also a little sore, but we were told that these could be good side effects—more evidence that his system was reacting to the treatment, instead of being unfazed by it.

Everyone's spirits were higher, and it was easier to stay positive during that round. The thought of going home was medicinal, too, and became Trey's main focus during the last part of August. He was no longer living in limbo, unsure of when he would return to familiar ground. Now he could see an actual departure date on the calendar and count down the days until he would run onto the football field again.

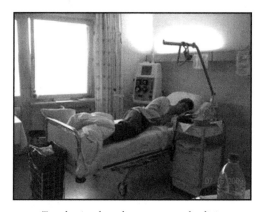

Trey sleeping through treatments at the clinic.

Trey worked out at the gym whenever he felt up to it and vowed to keep weight on despite the sugar-free diet. I had been making weekly trips to the market in the middle of Prien to buy fresh blueberries for Trey, filling up a picnic basket that probably held a couple of gallons. The first time I returned from the market after Trey learned we were going home, he ate the entire supply of blueberries in one day!

Charlie came back to Germany right after Ann left and we talked Trey into joining us for one last European adventure before heading home. This time, we made it a weekend excursion and headed to Bolzano, Italy, which was only a couple of hours away from Prien. Unfortunately, Charlie's history with European holiday travelers tried to repeat itself. Two hours turned into five as we crawled along the autobahn. I was driving, but because we sat still so much, I multi-tasked by finishing up a needlepoint project!

After spending some time driving lost and confused in Bolzano, we found a hotel with employees who spoke English, much to our relief. We then headed to the South Tyrol Museum of Archaeology to see "Otzi—the Iceman," a mummy promoted as the most well-known and important one in the world. The exhibit included a recreation of Otzi, formed by Dutch artists and based on what scientists believe he looked like while alive between 3350 and 3100 BC. No pun intended, but the Iceman was very cool to see, and even Trey was impressed.

We spent the night in Bolzano and splurged on a good dinner that Trey devoured, partly because he was hungry and partly because he was thinking about his football weight. The next day we took a drive down WeinStrasse, also known as Wine Road of Caldera. It wound up and around the Alps as it took us past hundreds of gorgeous grape and apple vineyards, one after the next. After a little roadside wine tasting and some incredible photo ops, we headed back to our temporary German home in Prien, where Trey was eager to start packing for the trip back to our real home in Georgia.

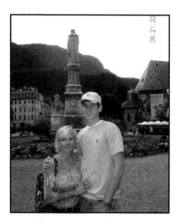

*Taking in the sights and tastes of Italy before heading home
to the United States in between treatments.*

Three days later, we were airborne, on our way back to family, friends, football, and what we hoped would be two weeks of Trey living life like the normal teenager he was determined to be. Unfortunately, Dr. Lentz wouldn't sign off on Trey playing in the game against North Forsyth. Initially, Charlie and I tried to convince Dr. Lentz of how important this game was to Trey. However, with the port having just been removed from Trey's chest, the possible consequences of a hard hit made it too risky to be out in the middle of all the action. It could cause a main artery to hemorrhage. Despite the medical warning, Trey didn't take the news very well. He was upset and deeply disappointed, but at least found some solace knowing he was on his way home, briefly free to join his teammates on the sidelines where there were no ports, IV needles, nor long hours connected to a machine.

The day we landed on our familiar Atlanta turf, Trey was bound and determined that the first stop would be the football field at West Forsyth High School. By the time we were off the plane, driving from the airport toward our home in Cumming, football practice was underway.

I'll never forget watching Trey walk down the silver-gray bleachers out onto the field where his teammates were warming up for practice. In one incredible moment, it seemed every player stopped what he was doing, turned and spotted Trey, and began clapping.

Hearing the applause and seeing the support this entire team had for Trey just about took my breath away. It could not have been more perfect if it had been planned and choreographed, but it was beautiful in its spontaneity.

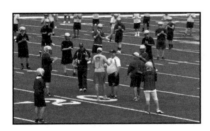

Trey's first visit to the football field after returning home from Europe.

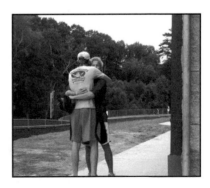

Trey gets a big hug from friend David Rooney.

From the heart, it was a genuine expression of how these guys felt seeing our Trey return to the fold.

There was really no point in trying to hold back tears as I watched from the main level of the stadium. For once, I didn't want to hold them back. These were true tears of happiness. I just let them roll.

Chapter Nine

Charlie

August 28, 2009. It had been less than three months since Trey received the news that his melanoma was back as stage IV. Cherie and I watched him do something that many might not have expected to see, given the gravity of his illness and the distance he was traveling to get his treatments.

We watched him run back onto the football field at West Forsyth, dressed in full pads and his blue number five jersey. August 28 was the first game of their senior year, and the one that had kept Trey motivated during long days in Germany. Determined to be here for it, he'd done exactly what he set out to do. Cherie and I were definitely experiencing a "proud parent" moment. Mostly, we were just happy. Trey had played the game for so many years, training hard and improving the way he performed in his position. He had earned the right to start his senior season on the field with his teammates, and it was good to see him out there where he was supposed to be.

Dr. Lentz had put limits on the trip home, though. Trey was cleared to return to the football field, but wasn't cleared to actually play in the game because he needed time for the catheter line to clot. Learning that he would be confined to the sidelines didn't please Trey, but he resigned himself to the doctor's orders. Considering the health battle he was facing, just getting to the sidelines was a pretty amazing feat.

Apparently a lot of other people thought the same thing. Trey was in no way expecting the support awaiting him in the stadium that night. West Forsyth's stadium holds about six thousand people, and it looked like every seat was taken for this highly anticipated game. Many of the fans, though, weren't dressed in the typical spirit wear you see at high school games. Instead, they were wearing "Play for Trey" T-shirts that the West Forsyth Touchdown Club had made, with Trey's jersey number and the date imprinted on them. The game, it turned out, was dedicated to Trey. The many shirts we saw throughout the stadium were testimony to how many people were pulling for him. The shirts were also a fundraiser sponsored by the club, with proceeds going toward his medical expenses. Like all other supportive measures, this was humbling and so appreciated—and a little mind-boggling when we realized that some people wearing the T-shirts didn't even know us personally.

The printed football program for the game also honored Trey by featuring him on the cover, which was created by a fellow West Forsyth teammate with a knack for graphic design. He took two separate pictures and blended them into one, coming up with a cover photo of Trey running with the ball while being uplifted in prayer by a circle of praying teammates. It was, and still is, known as the "Pray for Trey" cover.

WFHS football program cover from the West–North game.

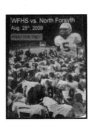

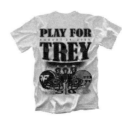

WFHS football T-shirts being sold at the game to raise funds for Trey's treatments.

This was the third year that West Forsyth played North Forsyth in football. As was tradition for all home games, the West Forsyth cheerleaders made a large sign for the football players to break through as they ran onto the field before kickoff. The sign this night acknowledged the third season of rivalry by saying "Round Three," but "Three" was crossed out with a huge X and replaced with "Trey." Of course, it was a play on Trey's name (which means three), so this was very clever and also a nice "welcome home" for our son.

His teammates insisted that he lead the pack by being the first one to run through it. Though Trey has had a lot of great moments on the football field, he was never one who gloated in the glory. So coming through the sign, high-stepping with his hands raised, was a genuine expression of how truly grateful he was to be back on the field with all the guys that night. The moment brought the crowd to its feet, and the cheers and bleacher-stomping shook the stadium like a freight train barreling through. The energy from excited fans was enough electricity to power on the Friday night lights towering above the field.

Atlanta news stations came out to report on Trey's return to the field. He also had a pre-game radio interview on Sports Radio 680 "The Fan" with John Kincade of the Buck and Kincade show, which is the longest running sports show in Atlanta history. The coverage was astounding, and made us realize how much Trey's story was really spreading outside of our small community. There had always been a little media coverage about his fight with melanoma, but interest gained a lot of momentum after the cancer returned, and we were seeking an alternative treatment plan.

This night, though, wasn't about cancer or treatments. It was about a football game and a team that had all its players run onto the field. After a long summer of just hearing about what was happening with his Wolverines, Trey was physically present to be part of the story. It was what he had aimed for all summer, and his attitude toward achieving that goal was the same attitude he applied to fighting cancer. God willing, it was going to happen.

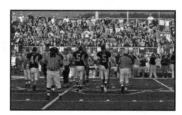

Trey (#5) walking across the field as one of the night's team captains.

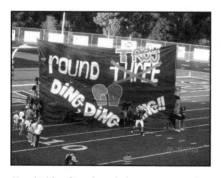

Trey (#5) breaking through the sign on game day.

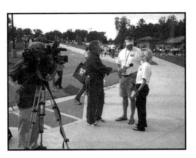

Charlie and Cherie speak with Atlanta news
reporters outside the West Forsyth High
School stadium pre-game.

Trey

Germany was as far from my mind as its literal distance in miles from my home when I walked into the locker room for the first time since spring. Putting on my uniform and equipment was like getting back into a favorite pair of pajamas—so comfortable and natural— and something I had really missed. If I'd ever before complained about wearing full pads in the heat and humidity of Georgia in August, I didn't now. Guys have quit football teams over stuff like that, but when you miss out on something for a while, you realize that some discomforts really aren't that big of a deal. Besides, after spending the summer with a line in my chest, switching to football pads was a relief. I was so glad to go back to school too. That's another thing I might not have looked forward to before melanoma, but you start appreciating the routines of your life when they're broken by something like cancer or another disease. I was in good shape with the classes I'd taken up to my senior year, and my counselor Bob Carnaroli had worked out a schedule through the school's online network that let me work remotely while in Germany. My teachers posted the same assignments everyone at home was working on. When I got back and returned to an actual classroom, I was at the same place everyone else was, so staying caught up was pretty easy.

I was scheduled to go back to Germany on September 13. Dread doesn't begin to cover how I felt about that upcoming trip, but I tried to think of it as one more hurdle to knock down on the road back to normal. I also tried to focus on the present and enjoy every day I had at home—seeing my friends, driving my truck on familiar roads, and dressing for football practice even though I wasn't medically cleared to play . . . yet. I believed there would be more trips home, and that I'd play some time during my senior season.

A lot of my friends were talking about college applications and preparing to submit them. I'd been thinking about them, too, and realized that I probably wouldn't continue playing football past high school. Several universities had been recruiting me junior year, but stopped calling after I got sick again. Only the University of West Georgia had stayed in contact and was still willing to give me a chance. They were also talking to my friend Nathan, so that was a plus, but I was really starting to think that my last high school game would be my last one. Period. You can have a great experience with a sport or hobby, but that doesn't mean it's something you do your whole life. The lessons learned from it will always stay with you, but the activity itself might only be temporary. Maybe that's what football was for me. I had always wanted to go to the University of Georgia, even though I knew I wouldn't play for them. They became my first choice for college applications.

Even though I was starting to recognize that college football might not be in the cards, my passion for high school football never waned. If anything, I was more fired up than ever, accepting that this might be my last playing season.

Before we even left for the second trip to Germany, I was already looking ahead to another break and wondering which game it would coincide with. I knew I had to get home again, and next time, I was going to be cleared to play. There just wasn't any other choice.

Cherie

Those two weeks home were like a vacation from the present to the past. Charlie, Trey, Wes, and I easily slipped into what felt like old times, with the house lit up as friends stopped by after the West–North Forsyth game. This had long been a normal occurrence at our house after home games. Sometimes we ordered pizza, and sometimes Charlie took something amazing out of the smoker that he had been tenderly babysitting all day. Trey and Wes were always surrounded by friends, and their friends' parents would often visit with us too. Somebody in the crowd always videotaped the game, and it would get reviewed and scrutinized late into the night. These were good times.

The North Forsyth Raiders broke a two-year losing streak, beating us thirty-seven to zero. I hated that for the boys who had practiced so hard, but there just wasn't much that could bring my high spirits down that night. My family of four was together again, all under the same roof for the first time in months. I knew a return to Germany was in the not-too-distant future, and was thankful the option was there for us, but Dorothy was right when she said, "There's no place like home" in *The Wizard of Oz*. I was completely wrapped in that feeling.

Dr. Lentz had arranged for Trey to undergo CT and PET scans in Atlanta on September 9. We were hopeful they would show more progress from his second round of treatment, and couldn't let our minds wander to thoughts of poor results. I just couldn't entertain the idea that we had gone to Germany for nothing.

The timing of the trip, the way it quickly came together, all the prayers that followed us overseas, and the fact that it felt right to me the minute we set foot inside the clinic— all of this convinced me that we were doing the right thing for Trey.

His test results in Atlanta seemed to confirm it, showing that there had been no growth of the tumor in Trey's left lung and no cancer developing anywhere else in his body! Results also confirmed the presence of "necrosis" in the lung tumor, which is the medical term for dead tissue within it. The deadly cancer appeared to be dying off.

Dr. Rapkin, Trey's Atlanta oncologist, saw the test results and took a neutral stance on the treatment in Germany. Whether it was his medical opinion or more about liability concerns, he wouldn't validate us continuing to forego traditional recommendations. However, he didn't discourage us from moving forward with the treatment, either. We accepted this as good news and confirmation that the treatment in Germany was showing signs of success. Three days later, we returned to Germany, hoping and praying that more small victories would come our way.

Chapter Ten

Cherie

Our second trip to Germany was easier for Charlie and me than the first one, since we knew our way around and were more familiar with local customs. The three of us were no longer living right on top of each other, either. We were able to rent a small house with more breathing room. Though very old and outdated in many ways, our rental offered a good and solid Internet connection. It was also nice to have the convenience of a kitchen, instead of relying on the hotel to warm food for us. The autumn weather was cooler, with temperatures averaging fifty-five to sixty-five degrees. This was a welcome change after the sweltering summer heat in a hotel with no air conditioning!

Our readjustment to Germany was especially made easier by the other families at the Lentz clinic. We reconnected with several American families from our first visit, but also befriended new arrivals from the United States and other countries. The support, empathy, and friendship that carried through this group of patients and their loved ones was tremendous. We began referring to the waiting area as our "Family Room." I realized how quickly bonds can form among people facing similar trials; we became very comfortable and trusting of each other. I even agreed to let the husband of a patient from Ireland perform acupuncture on my neck, shoulders, and back! He did the procedure right in the Family Room and brought great relief to the nagging pain I had been having in those areas—probably associated with the stress we were under.

Though Trey was receiving the same twelve-day treatment he had for the first and second rounds, he didn't experience any side effects during the third go of immunepheresis. This scared me at first, since the doctors had initially said the fever, chills, and other flu-like symptoms could be a positive sign that his system was responding. This time we were told that the lack of side effects might be a good sign, indicating that the cancer was limited and there was very little of it left for the immunepheresis to fight. I latched on to that possibility, even though it would be four or five weeks before Trey could have new scans.

Trey was grumpier than I expected him to be during this trip. Maybe the visit home had been too good, making it harder for him to readjust to Germany. He definitely did not want to be there, but I reminded him that we could and would get through this. Thankfully, friends back home had told us about TV streaming via Slingbox and arranged for us to access it, allowing Trey to keep up with sports on ESPN and watch college and NFL football games. Of course, the German time zone didn't coordinate at all with the clock back home. He was up all night watching TV, and sometimes didn't give in to sleep until six or seven in the morning. He had always used his daytime hours to sleep during weekday treatments, but now this up-all-night-sleep-all-day pattern spilled over into the weekends.

Charlie returned to the states after a couple of weeks, to catch Wesley's sporting events and take care of things at home. His mother, Jeanie, joined Trey and me in Germany. Though Trey was glad to see his "Neanie," we had a hard time convincing him to leave the house. He was more reluctant about venturing out than he had been during the summer. His outlook about recovery stayed optimistic, though, and he was looking forward to the next trip home, so I didn't worry that clinical depression was behind the sleep schedule and hermit-like existence. He simply had no interest in Germany or any part of Europe. Very little about this part of the world impressed him, not even the chance to ride the train to Munich and experience an authentic Oktoberfest. ESPN was his preferred entertainment, and it entertained him plenty.

Trey's third round of immunepheresis would be followed by a longer break than before. Our plans were to head home in early October and stay until the first part of November. It just couldn't come fast enough.

Trey

I probably hated Germany more the second time than I did the first. I guess that's understandable, considering the reason I was there, but even today, I have no interest in visiting Europe even as a regular tourist. I have college friends who look for chances to study abroad in London, Paris, Rome, and other European cities, but I'd rather keep my academics on the American side of the Atlantic.

The two weeks at home went by way too fast. I had felt normal while I was home, but coming back to Germany was a reminder that I wasn't normal; I was seventeen and fighting a deadly disease. Mom was all about keeping things positive, and I'm thankful that she was, but I just wanted my first cancer-free day to hurry up and get there. Even though school had only really just started, I felt like I'd already missed out on too many memories of my senior year.

It was cool, though, how friends at home kept me in the loop at school. I found out that I'd been elected Homecoming King, and that Wes would stand in for me since I'd still be in Germany the weekend of the Homecoming game and dance. I smiled at the image of Wes wearing a crown and a sash, but the night of the game, Mom stuck a toy crown on my head to celebrate my new

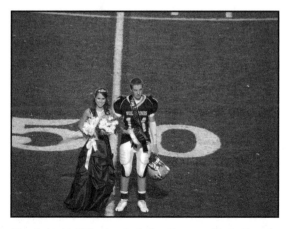

Wes, clad in his Wolverines football uniform, stood in for Trey who was named West Forsyth's 2009 homecoming king.

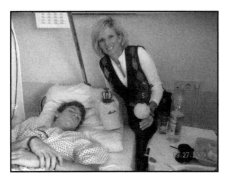

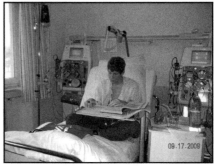

Cherie celebrates Trey's homecoming king honor with a small crown and homemade septor with the #5 painted on it during their stay in Germany.

Trey kept up with his school work to stay on track to graduate with his classmates.

royal title. It was hard not to appreciate the way she tried to make things a little easier.

We left for home on October 2, and this time I was cleared to play football! It looked like I could play right through West Forsyth's regular season before returning to Germany again. It was awesome letting my friends and coaches know I was coming back. Given the seriousness of melanoma stage IV, and the statistics you see about it, I know there were people who worried I might not be able to play football or do much of anything ever again. What a lot of them probably didn't realize is that football seemed to be what God used to help me stay focused and motivated, to keep moving forward instead of feeling sorry for myself. Football was my passion, so much so that the first thing I asked doctors when I learned the cancer was back was if I could play football that year.

I think the lessons learned from years of playing kicked in too. Perseverance and discipline are required to stick with this sport. I needed both of those to fight something that only had a five percent survival rate under traditional treatment. Teamwork is another part of football that counts for a lot. It's not a one-person sport; it takes everyone to make a touchdown happen. I had a lot of people helping me fight melanoma. The "Pray for Trey" Facebook page had over five thousand members at the time, and lots of those folks took the time to post encouraging messages. While in Germany, I got a letter from Vince Dooley, the University of Georgia's former head coach and athletic director, wishing me the best. I also got a couple of inspirational emails from the current head coach, Mark Richt. For someone who is a serious Georgia Bulldogs fan, hearing from those men was a huge deal. Their letters meant a lot to me and my family.

More and more people were asking for the "Pray for Trey" wristbands. We started hearing stories about how they were being spotted way beyond our community. Jeff Owens, a defensive tackle at UGA who had been coached in high school by our team's head coach, Frank Hepler, back in Florida, heard about me and asked for a wristband to wear in my honor. That blew my mind.

Mom said you don't always realize who you have in your life until they're highlighted. She compared them to angels around you that suddenly step forward when you need them the most. I had a lot of angels around me, from close friends to complete strangers. It made me feel better knowing that people were thinking about me and praying for me.

Michael Carvell, a reporter for the *Atlanta Journal-Constitution*, contacted my parents at some point for permission to run a story on me. Most of the interview was done over the phone in Cumming between trips to Germany, but later Mr. Carvell met me on the football field to expand on his story. The article was published on October 18—"Football Gives Him Hope in Cancer Battle." We talked about the good thoughts and prayers people were sending my way. My exact words to him were, "It's big . . . It's one of the most important things going for me in this process." That story connected us to so many people who wanted to help me in some sort of way: financially, through volunteer work, buying wristbands for their football teams, but most importantly, by sending prayers my way.

West Forsyth finished the football season 6–4, with some big wins and some painful losses. I suited up as safety and played almost every down for the rest of the season, looking for all the tackles and interceptions I could get. One of the biggest games was on October 23, against the Flowery Branch Falcons. It was a home game for us, with Flowery Branch (home of the Atlanta Falcons training camp) located about twenty miles from Cumming. Flowery Branch had a phenomenal team and we wanted the win so bad. It was one of those neck-and-neck fights right up until the bitter end, but

West Forsyth was ahead with less than a minute left on the scoreboard . . . when Flowery Branch threw a Hail Mary pass and won, fifty-four to fifty-one.

Man, that was a hard loss—except that Flowery Branch did something that made them even more phenomenal than they already were. After hearing about my fight with melanoma and how much the treatments in Germany were costing, members of their Touchdown Club started donating money to help cover some of the expenses. The whole campaign was headed up by Amy Todd, wife of Club President Andy Todd and mom of senior Falcon player Austin. They didn't even want credit for what they'd done, but West Forsyth's then-athletic director, Dennis Stromie, really thought they deserved recognition for their generosity. At halftime, right after the bands performed, the Todds met my parents at midfield and handed them an envelope containing $4,515 in cash. People in the stadium went so crazy cheering and applauding that some say they still get cold chills just remembering the moment. Amy Todd was quoted in the *Forsyth Newspaper*: "Athletic competition is great and wonderful, and we all love it, but when it comes to something like taking care of our kids, there are no opposing teams." I guess she summed up what the real spirit of community should be. I really liked that the Falcons team cared about my situation, but didn't go easy on me or treat me differently from any other player on the field. They brought an intense game of football, which is what I wanted.

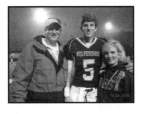

Charlie, Trey, and Cherie on West Forsyth High Senior Night.

A few weeks before it was time to go back to Germany, the high school chapter of the Fellowship of Christian Athletes held an event called "Fields of Faith." It was mainly supposed to be an on-campus night of music by contemporary Christian bands, which was pretty unusual in a public school.

The organizers asked me to speak about God's role in my fight against melanoma. I said I would, even though I'd be standing there in person talking to a large group instead of doing it over Skype. With the coaching and mentoring of Kevin Ragsdale from church and Coach Gary Sylvestri from West Forsyth, I felt like I could do it without getting too nervous. As it turned out, fifteen hundred students attended, the biggest crowd of people I had ever spoken to! It was a great experience for me to be part of—mainly because of what happened at the end of the night. Trying to show people what my life had been like during cancer treatment in Germany, and how God was the center of my world as I fought to get through everything, I made a two- or three-minute picture video that was set to the song "With Arms Wide Open" by Creed. Afterward, I looked out and saw about two hundred of my fellow students get up out of their seats, walking toward me. When they reached the stage area, they got down on their knees and accepted Christ into their hearts. I saw with my own eyes that, even though a bad thing like cancer had come into my life, God was highlighting the good things—in fact, about two hundred good things on just that one night.

In early November, I had more PET and CT scans at Egleston Children's Hospital. Obviously, we were hoping they would show that the tumor in my lung was gone or at least smaller, but that wasn't the case. My status was "unchanged" (or stable), but Dr. Lentz still thought I should come back to Germany for a fourth round of treatment. Mom reminded me that it was a good thing. I was still making progress with the treatment, but it was just going to be a longer road than we thought.

Charlie

The October 18 article in the *Atlanta Journal-Constitution* brought up the staggering cost of traveling to Germany for treatment. It mentioned, too, that I had been unable to find work after being laid off in the residential construction financing industry. Cherie, who had been in sales for twenty-one years with a private mortgage insurer, was seeing a real slowdown in business, but it was actually a blessing because it gave her the flexibility to always accompany Trey overseas.

With the alternative immunepheresis treatment alone running about eighty thousand dollars a month in Germany, and none of it covered by insurance, we were so grateful for the fundraising efforts in the community. Trey had missed the pancake breakfast and auction event held in August, but he did join in the "Tee Off for Trey" golf tournament before heading back to Germany for round four. Held at the Atlanta Country Club in Marietta and hosted by several friends of the Rood family, it included a silent auction and a cocktail and buffet reception. In total, the event raised a staggering sixty-five thousand dollars! We were really blessed to see so many friends, family members, and people Cherie knew from the mortgage business come out to support us, making sure that every player spot on the golf course was filled and that the silent auction was a huge success.

Cherie's sister Ann helped us connect with an organization called Helping Hands Ministries (HHM) in Tallulah Falls, Georgia, which could set up a fund for tax-deductible donations. HHM is a Christian-based foundation that formed to help those in situations similar to ours collect funds for care and expenses. Once again, Kevin Ragsdale stepped up to help us. He and our neighborhood friend Ashley Bartsch worked with Ann to get the fund established. There was also a "Holiday Bowl" football game and fair at West

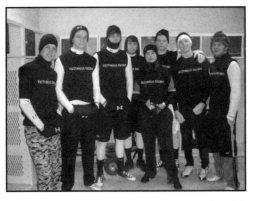

Trey's team "Victorious Secret" at the Holiday Bowl football game fundraiser.

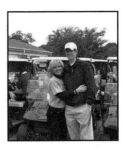

Cherie and Trey pause for a quick hug and pose at the "Tee Off for Trey" golf tournament.

Forsyth that Coach Hepler and his wife Heidi organized. A food tasting was another fundraiser held and sponsored by Nahm Thai Cuisine in Alpharetta, Georgia. All around us, people were coming up with creative ways to ease our financial burden.

Now we just had to keep trusting that the Germany plan was going to deliver the outcome we wanted. While the unchanged status of Trey's lung tumor was good in that the tumor hadn't grown, his scan results would have been more encouraging if the tumor had shrunk. As Trey began another round of treatment much like the earlier ones, Cherie asked Dr. Lentz about hitting the tumor harder by doing "around the clock treatments" for forty-eight to seventy-two hours at a time. She had previously addressed this option. She really felt like it might make a difference and was worth trying. She also knew that Trey was too beyond "done" to go through treatment any longer than he had to. The doctor said he had been thinking along those lines as well. Even though it was a very intense approach, he was comfortable that Trey was strong and healthy enough to take it. Cherie remained positive, believing that this aggressive approach would answer our prayers.

Chapter Eleven

Cherie

As a mother operating in survival mode, I wanted the timer on Trey's new treatment plan to start immediately. The unchanged status of Trey's tumor was not what I had hoped to see, and while I was determined to stay positive, I was getting anxious. I tried to hold tightly to the fact that Dr. Lentz had used this approach with two other patients and both were in remission, including one who had been stricken with a very rare form of breast cancer. Based on what we knew at the time, those patients also had multiple tumors to attack, whereas Trey only had one. I hung on to that knowledge as well.

Dr. Lentz had installed new immunepheresis machines several weeks earlier, but returned them to the manufacturer in Geneva to have a few adjustments made. Though he was hopeful that he could get some of the machines rushed back, he also needed some of his nurses to agree to work additional shifts. Fearing that the new plan would be delayed, I inquired if we could just employ the old machines Trey had used in prior rounds. He promised to think about it, but thought it would be much better to use the newer ones. So he would work to get them shipped back quickly.

For me, "quickly" meant having the new equipment back in time for Trey to begin our new protocol within a matter of days, but I realized that was wishful thinking in all likelihood. I asked if Dr. Lentz could extend the amount of time Trey spent on the older machines. Dr. Lentz replied that time could be extended on them, but intensity was already at the maximum. Still, I felt better that at least we could extend the time. Things would come together.

The weather was mostly cold and rainy, which only contributed to Trey's boredom and home sickness from the outset of this fourth trip. I had hoped that the new Xbox "Call of Duty" game would ease some of that, but we could only find the German-language version. God love him, Trey gave it the ol' college try, but it just wasn't playable in German!

He was encouraged about the new extended treatment plan, though. As he had been from the first day of his diagnosis, Trey was willing to go with whatever form this fight against melanoma took. Whether the "turbo treatment" ran for forty-eight hours, seventy-two hours, or somewhere in between, he loved that it meant this visit would be wrapped up much faster than usual—which, in turn, meant he'd be on a plane headed home all the sooner. The smile on my son's face told me he was just fine with this new plan.

On November 12, Dr. Lentz extended Trey's treatment time. I remember that it was a Thursday and he wanted to keep Trey on immunepheresis through Saturday—approximately sixty hours. I saw this as very good news, but was also keenly aware that it would be the definitive answer as to whether immunepheresis was going to work for Trey. Had our prayers been heard? Had all the positivity counted for anything?

The clinic was usually closed on weekends, but three nurses had agreed to rotate coverage through Saturday night. Bending the rules, I was allowed to stay as well, sleeping in a room next to Trey's. The accommodation was such a relief. Throughout the rounds of immunepheresis over the months, I had never spent a night away from my son. Doing so while his treatment was taking this more intensive turn would have been unbearable. (Not only for me, but for the nurses as well, since I probably would have been calling every half hour for an update!)

With medication to help him sleep, and dreams of the flight home always in mind, Trey adapted to the new protocol. Of course, he was given breaks throughout the duration, and would sometimes use them to check on me. The first night, he woke up at three-thirty a.m. and told the nurse on duty he needed to use the bathroom. Instead, he snuck away to peek in on me, double-checking that I was there. I'm pretty sure it was as important to him as it was to me that we not be separated.

Unlike during the daytime, the overnight hours at the clinic were very still and quiet. There were no families to pass the time with and none of the busyness of nurses tending to patients. I had a lot of time for just me and my thoughts, which I was actually able to reflect on with a glass of wine in my hand—something I'm sure I would have had to smuggle into an American clinic!

Germany, I realized, had been a time of hard life lessons about learning to be patient and holding firmly to your faith. It had meant months of maintaining positive expectations while balancing being prepared for whatever negative news might be delivered. Accepting that we were on a journey that didn't seem to follow any rules, I wondered if I had developed a thick enough skin or a strong enough faith to endure any- and everything from here on out.

Two days after Trey's new treatment ended, we were on a plane to Georgia. Two weeks after that, test results showed that Trey's tumor remained "unchanged" or "hard to call."

What now? The truth was, we didn't know the answer. We could only ask for prayers, wisdom, and direction as we headed into the holidays, a season we decided would best be used as a time of rest and renewal. We would give ourselves a short break from dealing with cancer by surrounding ourselves with family, friends, and the comforts of home. January would arrive soon enough. That's when we would look at our options, which might mean reconsidering treatments we had passed on, staying on the current path for a while longer, or discovering opportunities we weren't yet aware of.

For the time being, we decorated a Christmas tree, planned good times of celebration, and cheered Trey on as he played in the first annual Rotary Bowl on December 19. Rotary Bowl is a football game featuring seniors from area high schools, hand-selected by their coaches. Trey was honored as Defensive MVP of the Rotary Bowl, with two interceptions and a game-changing touchdown-saving tackle, as well as named to All-County Football for 2009. His high school football career wrapped up with Coach Hepler describing him to the *Forsyth County News* as the "most courageous player I have been around. He is a fighter. He went through so much this year fighting

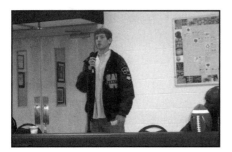

Trey speaks to peers and coaches at the Rotary Bowl banquet the night before the game.

Friends Ben Sasser and Cailin Mace pose with Trey after he was named MVP of the Rotary Bowl.

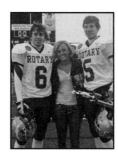

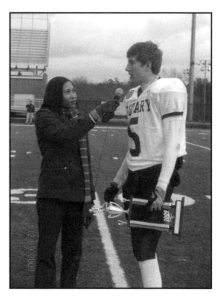

Trey gives a post-game interview with a news reporter at the Rotary Bowl.

melanoma and he still was a force when he was on the field." Not bad for someone who missed his summer practices.

We ended the holidays traveling to Colorado for a family ski trip in Steamboat Springs. This was a Make-A-Wish trip Trey had been granted from the Aflac Cancer Center. Qualifications included a cancer diagnosis prior to age eighteen, which Trey certainly met. Even though we had been encouraged many times to apply for this trip and just enjoy it, I was hesitant. I didn't want to take anything away from another child that might need a trip worse than our family. We had already been blessed with so much from other donations. I had always heard of trips or wishes granted for sick children who might not get the experience otherwise. My mind kept telling me that Trey would be okay, that this would not be his last chance to go on a trip, and we would be back to normal life at some point. However, so many friends and family encouraged us to take it, including the social worker at Aflac Cancer Center. I finally relented. Trey really wanted to go. Realizing that it was another chance for him to feel normal, I started looking forward to it too. It was so nice to pack for a trip that didn't involve cancer treatments!

Breckinridge, Colorado, was a winter wonderland. This trip proved Trey to be as active on the slopes as he had ever been, brimming with an energy that seemed to match that of his brother and cousins. Watching him glide and swoop down and across the white hills, I grappled to understand how a strong, active, and healthy-looking young man like Trey could be burdened with a cancerous tumor in his lung.

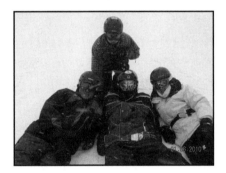

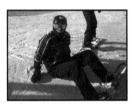

Trey with his snowboard in Breckinridge, Colorado for New Year's (2010).

Trey between Charlie and Cherie with Wes behind them on the ski slopes in Breckinridge, Colorado for New Year's (2010).

I imagine everyone who knew Trey's story wondered too. He certainly didn't look sick, nor did he act like it. Except when speaking to specific groups, like the kids at church, he rarely talked about his melanoma and tended to downplay it. If Trey wanted to stand out for anything, it was for what he did on the football field instead of what happened in a cancer clinic. Yet, he was sick—he was very sick, and we needed to continue finding a way to change that. When our holiday hiatus ended, the mission to find the way resumed, beginning with another set of scans in mid-January.

Our plans to move forward were instantly battered with a setback when the scans revealed two new tumors. Skeletal tumors. One was in Trey's ribs, while the other had staked its claim in his right lung. How?

They weren't even present a few weeks earlier, but now they were blatant.

Trey's stage IV cancer had never gone away, so this wasn't like getting the devastating news that it had returned. This was terrifying news that the cancer had no intentions of leaving. My questions about the power of prayer and positivity seemed to have been answered, and the answer appeared to be "no"—they had not made any difference at all. Still, when people asked me what they could do for us, my only answer was to pray for us.

"We've been praying," was their usual reply.

"Just keep praying." It was all I could ask for!

I wasn't ready to give up on prayer and positive thinking. I wasn't ready to give up on anything, especially my son.

Supported by family and friends who agreed with us, Charlie and I couldn't accept that the disease was on the brink of a swift rampage, one that would end by proving to be true to its terminal reputation. We would not resign ourselves to palliative care treatment as the melanoma showed no mercy in claiming Trey. We would not devote the next few months to long goodbyes. Instead, we took active steps to change the game plan again.

Looking back, I realized that we had been changing the game plan ever since Trey's cancer had returned as stage IV. When doctors told us that the standard and recommended treatment offered a five percent chance of survival, all Charlie and I heard was that it gave us a ninety-five percent chance of losing our oldest child. As Charlie said, those odds were unacceptable.

We had said no to tradition and opted for the alternative treatment in Germany, which now had all appearances of a failure. Yet, we had to believe that it had helped slow down the growth of Trey's tumors. After all, he was eight months out with a disease that often took people much sooner with cruel and vicious tenacity. His body mocked the disease, carrying him through football and a ski trip, with a strength and quality of life that was better than what some healthy people had. The treatment in Germany had carried us to this point. Though it hadn't been the cure we hoped for, our son was still with us despite statistics that said he shouldn't be.

We didn't believe the immunepheresis was five months of wasted effort, and we were totally against thinking that Trey's days were numbered. Though we were at a point where some folks might accept what they believe to be an inevitable end, we couldn't sink into such resignation. For us, that felt like the easy way out—and it didn't sit right with Trey's mentality or his spirit. It couldn't define any members of his support team, either.

Trey was now facing a tougher game, but that didn't mean it couldn't be won. It just meant he needed a new plan, and with it, a new hope.

PART II

Chapter Twelve

Trey

I don't like to say my treatment in Germany was a failure. I guess some people think of it that way, since I didn't come home cured. You have to remember, though: advanced melanoma is a fast-growing type of cancer, but I went the entire fall with no new growth. That had to make those trips to Germany count for something.

When the cancer first came back as stage IV, I wasn't old enough for the melanoma clinical trials that were going on in the United States. In mid-January, when we knew for sure that we'd have to attack with a new plan of action, I was only a few weeks away from my eighteenth birthday. That made me old enough for the trials, and there were several to investigate. I knew the timing was a "God thing," and this showed me that He is obviously organized in everything He does.

I went back to school in January with everyone else at West Forsyth. My parents had always let me live life as normally as possible when I was home and not off getting treatment somewhere. I know they were worried about me all the time, but they knew not to try to lock me in a plastic bubble. I needed to feel like a normal high school student. Being kept away from friends wouldn't have helped me at all. Friends, teachers, coaches, and others in my community also played a big part in keeping me positive.

Nobody, though, was more positive than Mom. If any news about my condition shook her, she didn't show it to me. She was in a zone and just kept moving toward the next step, even if she didn't know what that was. She was sure there was something, and if anyone was going to find it, I knew it would be her.

She and Dad were checking into a lot of trial options. Among others, they were following leads to Dana-Farber Cancer Institute in Boston, Memorial Sloan-Kettering Cancer Center in New York City, MD Anderson Cancer Center in Houston, and anywhere else in the country that might be doing some kind of research on stage IV melanoma cancer. As good as it was being home and back in school, I was pretty sure I wouldn't be staying there much longer.

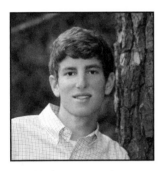

Trey's senior year photo.

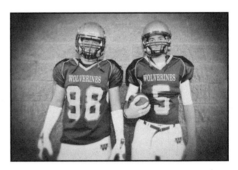

Trey had a series of senior portraits made including some with his friend and teammate Dustin Gayton (#98).

Cherie

Charlie and I had our moments of fear and despair after Trey's January scan results, followed by Dr. Lentz sadly telling us there would be no benefit in returning to Germany, but we couldn't stay in those moments for very long. Trey's cancer was no longer hibernating. By all indications, it had reawakened and was coming out swinging. We had to fight what was there and prevent more tumors from showing up. The question was, where did we go from here?

We started with a visit to Trey's oncologist Dr. David Lawson at the Emory/Winship Cancer Institute in Atlanta. After having turned down their recommended treatment in July, it was somewhat humbling to walk back into their offices asking for help, but thankfully, nobody berated us for traveling to Germany. Charlie and I, trying to make sense and find purpose out of the whole alternative treatment experience, didn't need people reminding us that the results were far from what we hoped for. The scan results had made that completely and frighteningly clear.

Back with Emory/Winship also meant we were back to looking at the intense IL-2 treatments we had hoped Trey wouldn't have to experience. The doctors hadn't changed their stance on this as the best approach for Trey. With nothing else on the table, we scheduled him to start treatment on February 15, 2010.

Meanwhile, we were looking at clinical trial opportunities for Trey. One of the first things we learned about the clinical trial process is that patients and their families have to self-refer all the way. Maybe it's because of liability concerns, but it seems like many doctors with a traditional treatment plan won't suggest trial options, leaving patients to search for, study, and pursue them on their own. When we started our research, we quickly saw how important it is for patients to realize that they might have alternatives to standard treatments—especially those treatments that have low success rates or are believed to be the last hope for a cure. There could be more possibilities out there, but people first have to do the legwork to find out that they even exist. I spent hours online reading through other patients' blogs, comments, and frustrations. I knew I had to learn, and learn quickly, what questions to ask and how to find the right people to talk to. After uncovering that the most productive talks would be with research nurses at melanoma research centers, I sought out any and all willing to speak with me. With the disease closing in on us and limited time, my phone calls were rooted in a deep urgency. People in the world of melanoma who picked up on my desperation were always quick to respond.

We were really encouraged by what we learned about the treatments and trials going on at the University of Texas MD Anderson Cancer Center, which is home to one of the largest melanoma and skin cancer programs in the world. The Ben Love/El Paso Corporation Melanoma and Skin Center was using the most advanced and innovative treatments and diagnostics for every type and stage of the disease.

For us, the most exciting news was that MD Anderson's nationally recognized research program was holding many trials for melanoma. They had also developed two promising melanoma treatments inside of a year, which was very impressive, given that there had been no real success anywhere else in a decade. We were eager to meet Dr. Patrick Hwu, Chair of the Melanoma Department and one of the leading tumor immunologists in the nation. We read that his clinical and laboratory work had led to advances in understanding the interaction between tumors and the immune system. He was credited as being a powerful force in the development of T-cell therapies, cellular immunotherapies, and other melanoma treatments we wanted to learn more about.

It was impossible to read about the highly regarded Dr. Hwu and not feel a burst of real hope. Of course, we wanted to talk to him about helping our son! Expecting a wait time of several weeks, I called MD Anderson on January 28 to make an appointment for Trey, only to find that they could schedule his visit February 2–5. It felt like an affirmation that we were going in the right direction. I wanted to believe that MD Anderson coming into the picture was turning out to be part of God's obviously organized plan for Trey's recovery.

Charlie and I delicately put together a timeline outlining Trey's journey so far with melanoma. Highlighting it with bullet points, we made a list any oncologist in the melanoma world could read and quickly understand our son's history with this awful diagnosis. It was hard to put it down on paper, but we included all treatments and occurrences from the day we first learned that melanoma had become part of our lives.

After talking to one of the research nurses in MD Anderson's melanoma department, and emailing her Trey's timeline, it was not more than a half hour before Dr. Hwu himself called us! Reaching out to us so personally and showing immediate interest in Trey's history was the affirmation that we had found our guy—someone who renewed our hope and filled us with excitement. This was the right plan of action.

Charlie

As Cherie said earlier, I collect and store information and trivia. That being something I can't deny, here are some facts about MD Anderson:

- In 2010, MD Anderson was ranked the top hospital for cancer care (for the fourth year in a row) in the "Best Hospitals" survey from *U.S. News & World Report.*
- Through donations, they've raised billions of dollars to support cancer research, patient care, education, and prevention.
- They rank first in the number of grants awarded from the National Cancer Institute.
- Since 1944, over nine hundred thousand cancer patients have visited MD Anderson for targeted therapies, surgery, chemotherapy, radiation, and proton therapy, immunotherapy, or combinations of treatments.
- The research program is considered one of the most productive efforts in the world aimed solely at cancer.

I did have some initial reservations about MD Anderson, though. My dad had been treated there during the 1980s. Even though a lot of years had passed since then, and research was more encouraging, I questioned if it really was our best choice. That is, until we dug deeper and compared it to other melanoma research centers. Cherie, unrelenting, called every single one in the nation, spoke to any research nurse she could get on the phone, and found out what Trey's options were. This was definitely a do-it-yourself venture.

Our appointment time arrived, and we were on our way to Houston. This was a trip to discover and learn everything we could about Dr. Hwu and his treatment recommendations for Trey. We not only found Dr. Hwu to be brilliant, but also encouraging, personable, and very likeable. Even with all the research notes and info we brought with us, you couldn't stump him or take him by surprise. He knew every melanoma doctor and treatment under the sun, and could explain in amazing detail the answer to any question we put in front of him. It was impossible not to be impressed. This gave us that "gut feeling" assurance that we were in the right place, and that God had once again led us in a good direction.

Dr. Hwu went over some of the trial options that Trey might be a good candidate for, but agreed with his Atlanta oncologist, Dr. Lawson, that the IL-2 regime needed to be completed first. We had to eliminate this standard treatment before moving on to other options. Even though it sounded like it could be a pretty rough treatment, and the Internet was full of stories about some pretty scary side effects, we learned that it was the game plan Trey needed to start with.

Though the doctors did some of the preliminary tests for the IL-2 during that visit to MD Anderson, Trey was still on course to undergo treatment in Atlanta on February 15. The expected routine was five or six days in the hospital (including the possibility of time in ICU), home for a couple of weeks, and back to the hospital to start over again. In early April, Trey would get scans to see where things stood, with the hope being that the IL-2 would eliminate any need to return to Houston and qualify for a trial.

As we headed to the Houston airport to catch our flight back to Atlanta, Trey did seem a little anxious about the IL-2 treatments. Throughout this whole fight with melanoma, he hadn't suffered any severe side effects yet, but IL-2 came with the threat of changing that. By the time we landed in Atlanta, his anxiety seemed secondary to his usual it-is-what-it-is resolve to do whatever it took to eradicate this thing from his life. Besides, he was on the ground and safely home, where plans with friends were under way. It was Friday, February 5—the beginning of Super Bowl Weekend.

Chapter Thirteen

Cherie

"Mom, I can't see!"

Less than twenty-four hours after returning home from Houston, I heard Trey shout those words from upstairs. Heart pounding, I hurried to his bedroom to find him stumbling about, trying to gain his bearings against the loss of his right peripheral vision in both eyes. As we made our way downstairs, his fear and frustration—edged with a little anger—was evident as he slammed one fist against the wall, as if to say *What now?* I understood his actions, because I was wondering the same thing.

My mind didn't automatically default to cancer being the culprit behind Trey's partial blindness. After all, he had undergone a full-body PET scan three weeks earlier. There were no signs that the melanoma had advanced to Trey's eyes, sinuses, or brain. Having recovered from meningitis that temporarily dimmed my own vision a year earlier, I knew that something else could be behind Trey's sudden loss of sight. He was also complaining of a slight headache, so maybe a migraine was coming on, or he was having side effects from those tests and scans. Whatever was going on, I was much too hopeful from the PET scan results to even consider that the cancer had spread to his brain. The PET scan had searched Trey from head to toe and would have detected any active cancer. Since it had found none, I was sure the vision issue had to be caused by something else.

Charlie and I drove Trey over to the home of our friend and neighbor, Dr. David Smith, who worked in the emergency room of our local hospital, Northside-Forsyth. "What do you think?" I asked him as we sat at his kitchen table, while he carefully checked Trey's eyes, ears, and vitals. Obviously, David couldn't make a diagnosis in his kitchen, but we hoped he could narrow down the possibilities.

The eyes, windows of the soul, can reveal the truth without any words. David's eyes said it all as he phoned colleagues at the emergency room. We were on our way, he told them, and Trey would need a brain MRI.

Trey

A walnut. That's about the size each of the tumors in my brain were. There were two of them, and they were side by side, in the back left hemisphere of my brain, though everything they were messing up was in the front. Going to bed with normal vision and waking up partially blind was not only scary, but also very frustrating. I mean, when was all of this going to end? I really had no doubt that it would end; I just wanted to know when. After rolling out of bed that Saturday morning, February 6, I never expected to be walking into walls. I'd hit another roadblock. First the Germany treatments didn't cure me, and now this.

My parents drove me to Northside-Forsyth where scans picked up the tumor. The news hit me like the worst football tackle I'd ever felt—times ten. This time there was no holding back the tears. Even Mom, who was always so determined to stay strong and positive in front of me, finally hit the point of falling apart. It was a real blow, and one we so didn't see coming. All I could think was, "Not another game plan changer." None of us had any clue what the new plan would be, much less what these new tumors meant for me. We just knew it was bad and that we were terrified.

Northside-Forsyth transferred me to Emory in Atlanta. Dr. Hwu told us to contact him if anything came up and to not start any kind of treatment except the planned IL-2 treatments without talking to him first. Anything we did in Atlanta might affect what he might want to do later in Houston. As it turned out, the brain tumors meant I'd be back in front of him sooner than I'd thought. After my parents called him with this latest news, we agreed that he would be my oncologist, and that all treatments from that moment on would be done at MD Anderson in Houston. Emory admitted me, but it was only to keep an eye on me for a few days and make sure I was stable enough to handle a flight to Houston. The biggest concern was that the tumors would cause me to have a seizure. I guess the changes in altitude and the cabin pressure inside a plane increases the chance of that happening.

I spent Super Bowl Sunday in the hospital with partial blindness in both eyes, which might have been depressing had I not had the greatest friends anyone could ask for. They pretty much kept me surrounded all weekend, possibly breaking the record for the most people in one hospital room at Emory. We all watched the Indianapolis Colts play the New Orleans Saints, which kept my strength and spirits up.

It wasn't the Super Bowl weekend we had been planning, but it was still a party, as well as a send-off since I'd be leaving for Houston the next day. I didn't want to go, but considering what was happening to me, I was glad we had somewhere to go and that nobody was saying there was nothing left to do.

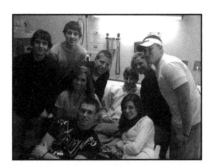

Super Bowl and send-off party at Emory
University Hospital in Atlanta.

Wes

The morning my brother woke up and couldn't really see, I knew Trey was in bad shape. Until then, I hadn't seen any major signs of how melanoma was tearing up his body. Watching him walk into walls and furniture was intense. It got very real, and I knew that he needed a miracle. I didn't know how to help, so I prayed and went to Facebook to post: "Pray for #5."

Once again, Mom and Dad were rushing around, making plans to take Trey out of town for treatment. At least this time they would all be staying in the country, which was comforting. I didn't want to go with them, though. Seeing Trey in a hospital bed bothered me too much. I didn't see him in one while in Germany, but just the pictures of him hooked up to that machine got to me. I was there for the Super Bowl game at Emory before he left for Houston, and it felt so unnatural to see him like that. My brother belonged on a football field or on the lake—not in a hospital bed with tubes and IVs stuck in him. It was hard to believe he had just been on the ski slopes at Breckinridge a month earlier.

Even after finding out the cancer had made it to his brain, Trey kept leading by example. He had a lot on his mind, but his attitude didn't turn sour at all. I saw him down some, but he never gave up. He was going to keep fighting just as he always had.

Cherie

Just like for the trip to Germany, Charlie, Trey, and I headed to Houston with little time to mull it over. Once again, we weren't exactly sure what we were getting into, but knew we needed to do it. One big difference, though, was that we now worried about Trey's ability to handle the flight. He hadn't had two brain tumors when we flew to Germany; the risk of seizures hadn't existed.

We were booked on a flight with Continental, which was an airline we didn't normally fly. I don't remember if it was boarding times, rates or what exactly made us decide on that particular flight, but we quickly realized it was the best one Trey could be on. As our flight attendant helped us get settled into our seats, he told us he had been formerly employed in the medical field and had a lot of experience working specifically with patients who had brain tumors. He was well versed in Trey's medications, and knew exactly what to do if a seizure happened. I could only see this reassuring man as another one of the angels put in our path.

Trey's vision hadn't improved any, but neither had it worsened. I'm sure he didn't like the loss of independence, but Charlie had to hold on to him some as we made our way through the Atlanta and Houston airports. In addition to the vision issues and seizure risks, we had concerns about him falling and hitting his head, which we feared might jeopardize him even more. Though he looked healthy on the outside, we knew he wasn't on the inside. Learning that two tumors had taken up residence in his brain made him seem so fragile, vulnerable to even slight injuries triggering a severe reaction.

We had not been at MD Anderson long before Dr. Hwu said two words we hoped to never hear: brain craniotomy. I think we knew we would hear them, but you're never prepared for how heavy and foreboding the words actually sound until they are being used in connection to your child. Trey's body had been through so much. Now they were making plans to remove a bone flap from his skull and literally touch his brain. At the same time, though, it was encouraging to know they could remove the tumors and hopefully restore his vision. Survival mode cranked up a few notches, as we told Dr. Hwu to do whatever needed to be done to stop the disease and save Trey's life.

Yet another new plan was developing. It included bringing another doctor on board. Dr. Syed Azeem was a neurosurgeon who would play a large role in Trey's vitality. All we could do was put deep trust in God and know we were in the right place—an incredible cancer institution where it was considered an honor to practice any kind of medicine. We were already investing a lot of trust in Dr. Hwu, so if Dr. Azeem was his choice for Trey's neurosurgeon, we were willing to move forward with confidence.

The surgery was scheduled for Friday, February 12. One of the pre-op routines was a visit to MD Anderson's Beauty & Barber Shop. Trey's head needed to be shaved. As always, he complied and accepted it as just another thing that needed to happen. In the three years since his first diagnosis, though, he had never lost a single strand of hair. Now he was going from a full head of hair to complete baldness. Had this been something a group of high school boys did to make life easier inside hot football helmets during summer practice, it probably would have amused me. When the reason is that your son is about to undergo brain surgery, it's hard to find something to smile about. Back home, though, family and friends were also shaving their heads in honor of Trey. The show of support really helped. It made us feel even more that people really were there with us in spirit.

The Beauty & Barber Shop was impressive. Just like many regular salons, it was bright and airy. It had licensed cosmetologists and fully equipped styling stations where patients could get shaves, shampoos, and haircuts, as well as pick out wigs, scarves, and hats. All the services are free, and many of the volunteers who work in the shop are cancer survivors themselves. Like everyone we met at MD Anderson, the folks in the salon were uplifting, compassionate, and made us hopefuls feel like we were in the right place.

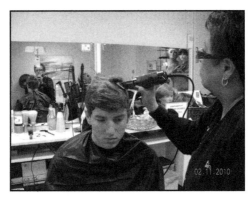

Trey getting his hair buzzed off to prep for brain surgery
at the MD Anderson Beauty and Barber Shop.

Waiting for the actual surgery date was tough. I knew I needed more support around me. Trey was about to undergo the most invasive surgery you can think of—brain surgery—and it was scary. Keeping the faith and thinking positive thoughts was nonnegotiable, but Charlie and I both needed others with us. We needed to get through this as a family.

I called my mom and asked her to come to Houston. Before I even finished making arrangements, my two best friends showed up like angels by special order, divinely sent. Rosie Stauber and Ginger Bowers arrived to hold me up on Trey's surgery day and through his recovery. They brought the gift of laughter, keeping our spirits up and Trey amused as they told funny stories, played games in his hospital room, and even managed to sneak some wine in for the adults. Mainly, they were there for support and to keep our minds from getting swallowed up by the fear and seriousness of what was really happening.

The day before surgery, Trey posted on Facebook:

The Lord our God, your God, my God . . . has an outstanding plan for each and every one of us. All you have to do is trust in Him with all your heart and believe in Him. Please pray for me. See you all soon!

That same night, Wes posted:

God, I just pray to you that everything works out tomorrow for my brother. I pray you give my family the strength to get through this. Give my brother the wisdom he needs. Keep his head up. Be with him and help him be the happiest he can be. Move Trey's mountain, God. I pray you give me the strength to stay strong. Give Trey the attitude he needs, God. You don't choose the qualified, but you qualify the chosen. That's awesome. I believe in that. I believe in you with all my heart. Move Trey's mountain, God. Be with him tomorrow as he goes through surgery. I believe in your plan. I love you God, I love you Jesus.

How could Charlie and I read those posts and not feel like we had been blessed with the best kids? We were proud that Trey's faith remained so strong in the face of what he was about to go through. We were proud of Wes and his love for his brother, and that whatever fears and concerns he had were being given over to the best possible resource.

"God things" were happening all around us, though, starting with our discovery that some friends from Atlanta who Charlie had known for years were at MD Anderson. Beth Jordan, accompanied by her husband Greg, was also there for brain surgery. During their back-and-forth visits, Greg had reconnected with an old high school friend named Bill Wade and his wife Christy. They only lived a few miles from MD Anderson and had a comfortable apartment above their garage.

The day before Trey's surgery, we were pleasantly surprised to get a hospital visit from Bill and his daughter Kylie, who was Trey's age. Though we were just meeting each other, the Wades insisted that Charlie use their apartment during this trip and any in the future. I always stayed in the hospital with Trey, keeping my promise to him that I would never leave his side—not that anyone could have pried me loose anyway! From that first visit with the Wades, a friendship blossomed between our families. Bill, Christy, Kylie, and their younger daughter McKinley always welcomed us into their home, sat with us during Trey's treatments, brought dinner, invited us to spend downtime with them, introduced us to some of their Houston friends, and always arranged a "special something" whenever we were in town. There is no doubt that God put them in our lives at a time when we needed giving and supportive friends like the ones we had at home. It was incredible to me that they would reach out to us—strangers, at first—and give so freely of their time. Since that first meeting, our friendship has only grown more wonderful, including some travels together. They are now some of our closest

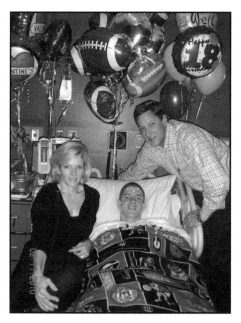

*Cherie, Trey, and Charlie the day before Trey's
brain surgery at MD Anderson.*

and dearest friends, the kind you are able to share so much of life with—good and bad.

Like so many of the earthly angels we seemed to be meeting along the road, the Wades walked into our lives with perfect timing—unannounced, but suddenly there at just the right moment. We were anxious and unsure of the outcome as we faced the first invasive treatment Trey would undergo since his original diagnosis. As we watched him being wheeled into surgery, we put our faith in those we trusted were sent by God. It had to be okay.

Chapter Fourteen

Trey

My brain surgery was called a success. The first question I had was: "When can I go home?" Sooner than you'd think. After getting moved out of ICU and into a regular room the next day, the doctors said I'd probably get to leave in about five days.

Mom told me funny stories about how goofy I was waking up from surgery and coming out of the heavy anesthesia. My head was wrapped in thick gauze, and I kept grabbing it and repeating, "I've been hit in the head by a rock" over and over again. I was so drugged that I had no idea what had happened at first. I knew I wanted Mom around all the time, but was so out of it that I mistook both Rosie and Ginger for her. Even under anesthesia, I guess I knew what special friends they are to Mom, and that's why I was so comfortable having them with me. Mom, of course, slept in the ICU room with me, and I knew she'd never leave my side. I don't think she thought anyone could take care of me like she could, and was always on the nurses for anything I needed.

To get to go home was something of a birthday present. The timing meant I'd be home with family and friends for my eighteenth birthday on February 19, 2010. Nobody would want to spend any birthday in the hospital, but this was a big deal because it still mattered a lot to me that I be in the mainstream with people my age. It had mattered back during football season my senior year, but seemed to take on an even bigger importance as graduation got closer. I still didn't want to be the guy who was seen as different from others his age, and being held in the hospital on your eighteenth birthday would definitely feel different.

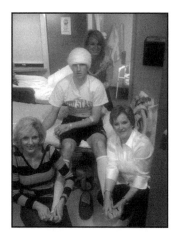 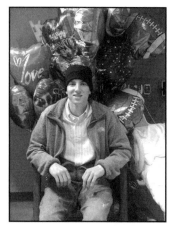

Fun and TLC from Cherie and family friends, Rosie Stauber and Ginger Bowers.

Trey is ready to return home following brain surgery—just in time for his 18th birthday!

I also knew it was going to be a short visit home. Dr. Hwu was just giving me a week's break before we'd return to Houston. I'd have the stitches taken out of my head, then receive gamma knife radiotherapy on the area where they had done the brain surgery. It's a form of radiation. They would also do radiation on another spot they'd found on the right side of my brain. After that, I'd have to start the IL-2 treatments, which I was seriously dreading.

My vision didn't miraculously come back right after the brain surgery, but we were still hopeful that it would. I really stayed upbeat about everything. I don't remember thinking I might not be able to drive again or do other normal things like reading or studying because of my eyesight. School hadn't been back in session too long from winter break before I ended up in Houston, but I still had the choice of taking classes online or showing up for them in person. People told me to go to school whenever I was "able to," but I was always able to go whenever I was home.

Mom asked that the prayer chains keep going and said we were going to beat this one way or another. I believed that more than ever when we got to

MD Anderson. The timing of when I ended up there—just when I was old enough to take part in trials—was too serendipitous for me to think it was random. Plus, from what I could tell at that point, they had more than one possibility for me. If something didn't work, there might be a plan B. For the time being, though, my first plan was to be home for my birthday.

Charlie

Trey's brain surgery took six intense hours. Cherie and I got updates every two hours. We were basically told that everything was going as planned and Trey was doing well. It was the best news we could hope for in those circumstances. I wanted to have the same high optimism that Cherie and Trey did, but these circumstances seemed to have come up so fast. I'd seen enough cancer in my immediate family to know the disease had an ability to return just when you were getting comfortable thinking that it might not. I'd already seen that happen with Trey, but also knew I couldn't get hung up on it. All of us had to stay positive, choosing the best option for Trey and refusing to let circumstances shake our faith and our will to keep going. Cherie's mindset would never give up. If a roadblock came along, she kept driving and looked for a way around it. Rosie and Ginger gave us all a lot of support during the surgery and the days that followed. I know it was important to Cherie for them to be there. As we went into this next leg of the trip, we were hoping the new plan at MD Anderson would be a clear path for Trey, leading to complete wellness.

Trey's surgery was on a Friday. We took him home the following Wednesday. His birthday fell that weekend, and Cherie and I did exactly what we would have done if cancer had never entered his life—we threw him an eighteenth birthday party. It was nothing crazy and elaborate, but was full of what he wanted: normalcy. Friends and neighbors streamed in for cake and all the usual celebrations, but there was one activity that stood out—a lot of Trey's friends shaved their heads, right there at the party, so they had the same buzzed look Trey had. The gesture was probably one of the best birthday presents I've ever seen.

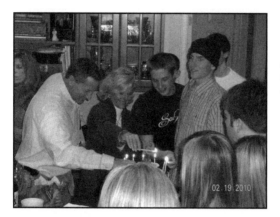

The family happily lights eighteen candles for Trey's birthday cake.

While our time at home went by fast, we really felt like we couldn't get back to Houston soon enough. Trey had found lumps under both armpits while we were home. That weighed on us as we flew back west, only to be joined by another scare after the plane landed. For about thirty minutes, Trey's vision was further marred by a huge black spot in front of his eyes. Early indications were that this return trip to MD Anderson was off to a rough start.

As it turned out, doctors suspected the flight itself caused the vision issue. Apparently, changes in altitude and air pressure spurred this unusual side effect of Trey's brain surgery, which put his hopes of returning home the weekend after gamma knife in jeopardy. Still, we were glad that's all it was. If the only treatment was spending a weekend in Houston, we were pretty sure we could deal with it.

We also got some hopeful news about the new lumps under his arms. The general surgeon who evaluated them was confident they didn't feel like melanoma, though he did still schedule an ultrasound to confirm they weren't. No matter what the results were, he said plans for Trey to begin IL-2 on March 8 were still on schedule.

Dr. Hwu also talked to us about an "insurance policy" in case the IL-2 didn't prove to be the right treatment for Trey. This insurance was actually a clinical trial Dr. Hwu was conducting. It was called "Lymphodepletion Plus Adoptive Cell Transfer With or Without Dendritic Cell Immunization in

Patients With Metastatic Melanoma." We called it "T-cell therapy" for short. The goal was to learn if dendritic cells made from special blood cells would improve the fighting ability of T-cells, or immune cells specific for melanoma. The blood cells and T-cells would be taken from the patient's blood and tissue, then grown in the lab before being inserted back into the blood. The research would also study if the cells could shrink or slow down the growth of metastatic melanoma when combined with IL-2 or chemotherapy.

Dr. Hwu had already talked to us about the trial, and had taken tissue from Trey's brain tumor to see if it would grow T-cells. The general surgeon believed they could also resect any other areas where there was tumor growing, such as the skeletal ones in Trey's right rib and shoulder. Though I'd had earlier reservations about MD Anderson being the right place for Trey, they were always showing us that they weren't going to ride on the hope of only one possible treatment for him. I was feeling good about them now, but, like Cherie, looked at the clinical trials as an "if" option. We were still hoping the IL-2 would be Trey's answer.

Next up, though, was the gamma knife radiation, which MD Anderson describes as "accurate tumor targeting with a single dose of radiation, freeing patients from multiple radiation treatments and allowing them to return to a normal routine within a few days of treatment." The doctors would focus a high dose of radiation on the exact dimensions of the surgical cavity where Trey's tumor had been. Mapping it out took a long time. The entire gamma knife process lasted fourteen hours. While the doctors were radiating the small right side spot, they found an additional spot lurking nearby. It was

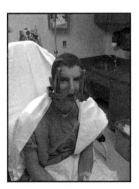

Trey donning the "Transformers" headgear (his nickname for it) in preparation for his fourteen-hour gamma knife radiation surgery.

tiny, but it was there—a huge reminder of what an aggressive disease we were dealing with.

Cherie

Charlie and I might have buckled under the stress of a fourteen-hour waiting game had it not been for the kindness of our new friends in Houston, the Wade family, as well as all of our friends and family back home.

Though it was a long sail, Trey came through the gamma knife radiation without any complications. As the detailed procedure promised, he was up for activity in a matter of days, but not the kind that appeals to anyone, much less to an eighteen-year-old high school senior. In the days leading up to the beginning of IL-2 treatment, Trey's time was jammed with X-rays, scans, lab work, and other tests—sometimes four or five in a single day.

It was a time of good news and bad news. The good news included confirmation that the lumps under Trey's arms were not melanoma, but likely side effects of the steroids and IVs from brain surgery. More good news was that his vision began to improve considerably, enough to actually impress the eye doctor! On the down side, we learned that tissue from his brain tumor had failed to grow T-cells, but even this news was cushioned with confidence that tissue from his skeletal tumors might be productive. There always seemed to be hope that something more could be done.

Trey's faith, strength, and attitude continued to amaze. I truly felt like there was no chance his medical ordeal could succeed in bringing him down or squelch his will to keep fighting. Where was the anger, bitterness, and question of Why me? If Trey wrestled with those feelings, he never expressed them. Even after all he had been through since 2007, his opinion remained firm that he would one day be done with melanoma, and every setback he faced was viewed as nothing more than part of the process toward recovery.

He was disappointed when the radiology oncologist nixed his hopes for going home the weekend before IL-2 treatments started. She felt like Trey was still at risk for developing side effects from the gamma knife radiation. I can't say I shared his disappointment because I was relieved to be staying in

Houston. The truth is, I felt safe when we were at MD Anderson, surrounded by people who were personally and medically involved and invested in saving my son's life.

Since Trey couldn't go home for the weekend, he was thrilled when someone from home came to see him. His friend Emily Pitts, a fellow West Forsyth senior, flew to Houston for the single purpose of visiting him. After a long week of grueling medical procedures, Trey got to be a normal teenager again. He took in a concert by country singer Jason Aldean, and attended a big Texas rodeo that was lively with bucking broncos, barrel racers, and clowns. I doubt that anyone who saw him, tall and easygoing as he moved about the crowd, thought for a minute he was a patient at MD Anderson. I couldn't believe it myself at times, because nothing about him said he was sick.

He was a face of melanoma, though, and word of his journey was beginning to spread beyond our local media. In March of that year, CNN commentator and host Nancy Grace picked up on Trey's fight and did a story about him on her show. Though it was short, she included some great pictures of Trey and graciously aired it multiple times, igniting a response from melanoma patients and supporters all over the country. Meanwhile, fundraising efforts were still underway for Trey, including the North Point Pediatrics "Jog for a Cause" 5K/10K in Alpharetta, Georgia. The event benefits various children and teens fighting cancer, and they selected Trey as one of the beneficiaries that year. About fifty friends signed up for Team Trey and took part in it.

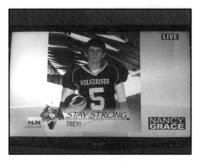

CNN's Nancy Grace picked up Trey's story (March 2010).

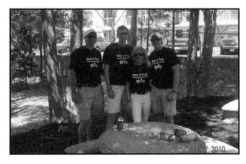

Charlie, Trey, Cherie, and Wes join the Ride-4-Trey motorcycle fundraiser.

Trey went into his IL-2 treatments with the prayers and support of so many people—a blend of close friends and family, classmates, neighbors, acquaintances, and strangers moved by his story.

The plan was for Trey to begin with a regimen of ten doses over a two-week period. The warnings about side effects proved not to be an exaggeration, with the scariest episode sending him into chills so violent that the bed shook. His heart rate shot up, and the quick palpitations forced the IL-2 to be called off after he was moved to ICU for treatment, observation, and recovery. While I had always known there was a chance the IL-2 might not work, it had never occurred to me that it could actually kill my son.

Surprising myself, I stayed cool during this episode, thinking, moving, and speaking with a strength I can't even explain. Perhaps it was another form of survival mode, of knowing that I would do Trey no good if I fell apart. Charlie had gone home to spend time with Wes, so it was just me witnessing Trey's crisis and telling the doctors and nurses to do whatever they had to do to save him. It wasn't like they needed my blessings, though, as they were rallying around him with such an intensity that anyone who didn't know the situation might wonder if they were overreacting.

Once Trey stabilized, he resumed the IL-2, completing the nine rounds without any more critical reactions. He did have severe chills, lots of water-weight gain, a red rash all over his arms, and some nausea. He also contracted an infection in part of his line, which caused a lot of pain and discomfort

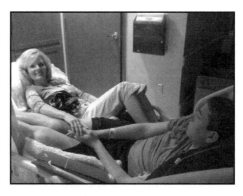

Cherie and Trey after Trey returned to his hospital room
following a trip to the ICU for treatment side effects.

until they changed his port to another location. Overall, though, Dr. Hwu was pleased with the way Trey handled the treatment and that his system was able to tolerate the number of doses administered within the time frame.

Trey was rewarded with a two-week break and went home, where he received the great news that he had been officially accepted at the University of Georgia, his dream school! I was one proud mom. The news of his acceptance to UGA was such an incredibly happy feeling. I remember when he called to tell me that his acceptance was posted on the university's website, I had him text me a picture of it. This really was one of those milestone moments when I remember exactly where I was as he told me. I was out with my sister Ann, having a glass of wine, and didn't even try to hold back the tears. These were happy tears, and after so many that had been spurred by fear, frustration, and sadness, these were welcome ones. Not only was I proud of and happy for Trey, but I understood what a huge deal this acceptance really was to him. Going to UGA was one of the targets Trey aimed for as he battled through melanoma, but before he'd know for sure, that target might have fallen through. Now it was real—he was in and could look at the bull's-eye as a sure thing waiting for him.

After we got this news, Trey's high school counselor, Bob Carnaroli (who had written an "incredible circumstance" recommendation letter when Trey applied), told us about the person in the UGA Admissions office who had played a key role in reviewing and approving the application. All I remember is that her name was Stephanie. I was overwhelmed with the desire to let her know what a gift she and her team had given Trey by welcoming him to attend their university. Without an appointment, I got in my car and made a special trip to the campus. I walked into the Admissions office and asked to see Stephanie, promising that I would only take a minute of her time.

Graciously, Stephanie agreed to see me. I don't think she expected to meet a bawling woman who had just dropped in to hug her! Despite the unusual way I introduced myself, we ended up enjoying a remarkable meeting that day, one I know we both walked away from feeling good about. I was also certain that she was another angel God had put in our path for Trey's sake and well-being.

Our euphoria about the future soon took a backseat to the present reality. Trey returned to Houston for another series of IL-2, following the same schedule he had before. This second series was a little easier on Trey. The doctors and nurses better knew what to anticipate based on his reaction during the first series. They were able to get ahead of some of the side effects, but we did have some delay when Trey developed a bad rash all over his body. After bringing in another medical specialist to diagnose the problem, we learned that Trey was having an allergic reaction to the antibiotic Bactrim. We had to wait for the rash to heal before completing the series, and the holdup was something that Trey really hated. He accepted, but never welcomed, news that he would need to stay in the hospital longer than expected, even though we were certainly used to the atmosphere. I tried to make the best of it by always toting along my three-inch Tempur-Pedic mattress pad, blanket, and pillow so that I could sleep in the standard pull-out chair found in whatever hospital room Trey was in. We usually arrived at the hospital with enough suitcases to look like people checking into an extended-stay hotel, but I tried to pack as many items as Trey might want. If any comfort of home could be crammed into a suitcase, I made sure it was.

The chills Trey experienced the second time proved to be worse than before, sometimes so intense that his bed literally shook and rattled with him. It was distressing to watch the chills take over and hear the metal bed frame banging against the wall. The nurses did a great job, armed and ready to cover him with warm blankets, which did help to bring the shivering under control. There were also some side effects from medication, but this time Trey didn't end up in the ICU, which was an improvement.

Since we were in the hospital's melanoma unit on the tenth floor, I spent a lot of time talking to patients in nearby rooms. They were going through similar treatments, so there were always people to share diagnoses and side-effect stories with. It is amazing what humans can bond and connect over!

When the second IL-2 series was behind him, Trey was given a three-week reprieve before undergoing tests to determine how well the treatment was working. Before leaving the hospital, he received a visit from Roger Clemens, former Cy Young Award-winning pitcher. One of Charlie's lifelong friends in Atlanta, Wes Pritchett, had arranged the visit. Wes had a contact in Houston who could get Roger to MD Anderson before we left for home. When he arrived, it was so cool that we were just "hanging out" with Roger Clemens! He made us feel so comfortable. He was interested in Trey, asking about his experiences playing baseball and other sports, and taking lots of photos with us. This was such a great moment for Trey, because he's such a big sports fan. Plus, Roger gave him Astros tickets to use the next time he was in Houston.

This next return to the home front found Trey thinking about other things, like ordering his cap and gown and getting fitted for a senior prom tuxedo. This trip home also coincided with spring break, but he really was too weak from the very recent IL-2 to go on the annual weeklong cruise with us and our neighborhood gang. Though missing the Caribbean sun was disappointing to me, I stayed on land with Trey, who was more than happy with his spring break alternative—attending the Masters Golf Tournament in Augusta and fishing on Lake Lanier with his dad and some friends.

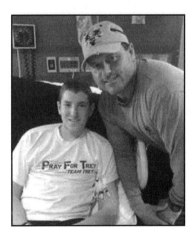

Trey receives a visit from Roger Clemens, legendary Cy Young Award-winning pitcher, at MD Anderson.

Trey looked great while he was home. Life was good, just the way I pictured it would always be before cancer struck and changed everything. Things that I had once taken for granted in life, I now viewed as milestones and blessings. What might have mattered a lot then now mattered very little, and what might have seemed little now seemed like a lot. We were soon back on a plane to Houston where Trey would get the results of his two series of IL-2 treatments. If he was showing progress, he would advance to a third round; if not, well, we weren't quite ready to think about that.

Once again, we were facing a combination of good news and bad news. The good news, Dr. Hwu stressed, was that Trey's brain MRI and chest/abdomen CT scans were free of new lesions or tumors. While the two small spots on the right side of Trey's brain showed increases in their size, he believed it was from normal bleeding out after the gamma knife radiation. Deep breath.

The bad news was that the CT scans also revealed the main tumor in Trey's left lung had grown slightly larger, as had a small upper nodule. The tumor on the right side of his rib had grown the most, but because Trey wasn't feeling any pain from it, Dr. Hwu was hopeful that it hadn't yet penetrated to the bone.

The bottom line was that IL-2 had not been successful. There was no point in moving on to the next series. Whether we were ready to think about it or not, there it was. It was time to look at plan B—a clinical trial. Hearing this, Trey brightened up and said, "My day just got better." Clearly, that might not be the expected answer from someone who had just learned his cancer treatments weren't working! Trey was happy not to deal with another wicked round of IL-2, though, and had faith that plan B—whatever it was—was a good option. "Don't forget," he reminded Charlie and me, "that God is on our side."

Chapter Fifteen

Trey

God was, and is, my hope. When I was first diagnosed in 2007, I couldn't say that God was first in my life. That had changed by the time I was looking at clinical trials in 2010. I remember crying one night and just saying, "I give my life to You. You're in control."

Browns Bridge Community Church used me in a video they made called "Why Bad Things Happen to Good People," where I gave a talk about what role I thought God had in all I had been dealing with. I talked about what I really believed, which was that I knew He had a plan and I had decided I would trust in it. Wherever it led me, wherever it went, I was going to accept it and go through each day believing that God was God. Whatever He had in mind for me would ultimately be best. The video is on the "Pray for Trey" Facebook page, but North Point Ministries (which Browns Bridge is a campus of) uses it for middle and high school programs on all five of their Atlanta-area campuses. I'm told, and I hope, that it's been a witness and message of hope to a lot of people.

I don't know what I would have done if I didn't have God to put my hope into. If He had been missing from my life, I think the melanoma fight would have driven me insane. Before 2010, my faith was building. That was good, because it started getting tested in a big way after we got home from Germany.

It's not that I was happy to find out that the IL-2 treatments hadn't worked. It's just that I was so relieved not to have to go through another series of what had to be the worst medical experience of my life. I would have been really discouraged if Dr. Hwu said MD Anderson had nothing else to offer me, but he didn't say that, or even come close to those words. Right away, he started talking about other possibilities. If God had brought me to MD Anderson—and I really believed He had—then I knew one of those other possibilities was my answer.

Just one month before I was supposed to graduate from high school, we started making plans to start with a trial that Mom, Dad, and Dr. Hwu thought was the best for me. It meant I'd have to go back to MD Anderson on May 10. It was the week after my senior prom, so I was happy with it. The way the trial was set up, I'd have a break around June 1—my high school graduation date. Once again, I could see that things from God aren't random. I knew I was on His timetable with all of this, but it seemed like He was really working with me on it.

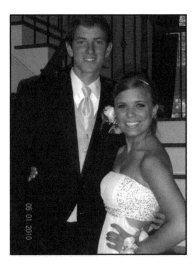

Trey and friend Emily Pitts attended West Forsyth's Senior Prom together.

Cherie

The trial Dr. Hwu wanted Charlie and me to consider for Trey was being conducted with Bristol Meyers-Squibb, a pharmaceutical company. It was a ninety-minute infusion of an antibody/immunotherapy drug called ipilimumab. Administered by IV, it was followed up five days later with the chemotherapy drug Temodar. The regimen wouldn't require a hospital stay, but would be carried out at four different times every three weeks, so that meant four rounds of this treatment. Over time, the span between treatments would be spread further apart.

Trey and I made the familiar trip back to Houston on May 10, so he could undergo all the scans and other testing needed to confirm that he definitely qualified to take part in the trial. The first requirement was that he be six weeks out of his last IL-2 treatment so that his liver enzymes and bilirubin, elevated from the infusions, would be back to normal levels. There was no medical reason to think that wouldn't happen naturally, since he was off the treatment. The bigger anxiety in all the pre-trial testing was what the brain scans would reveal. Hopefully, nothing new had developed and Trey would start the trial on May 12.

Then the plans came to a screeching halt. An MRI revealed five new melanoma spots on Trey's brain. Five. Even though they were small, they were still there. Dear God, it had only been two months since those were eradicated by the gamma knife radiation, and already more than twice as many had taken their place. This unrelenting and monstrous disease seemed determined to flex its muscles.

If Dr. Hwu could calm us with anything, it was the good probability that gamma knife would be effective in ridding Trey's brain of these cancerous spots as well. Because these were new spots and not a return of the original ones, we were hopeful that gamma knife would be the powerful ammunition to eliminate spots for good. This really was a war.

Trey's second gamma knife treatment would mean a twenty-one-day delay in being able to start the ipilimumab trial. We had no more resigned ourselves to the wait before more rough news swept over us. The radiology oncologist feared the five new tumors might be in the cerebrospinal (brain/spinal) fluid. If this was true, then the cancer had spread again.

We had not even been back at MD Anderson for three days, and the plan of action had changed twice as they charted a way to get ahead of the melanoma. To find out if it was in the cerebrospinal fluid, doctors would be putting Trey through a spinal MRI that late Friday, followed by a spinal tap early Monday, leaving us with an anxious wait-and-see weekend in between. Of course, they weren't doing this to be deliberately torturous. They were doing it because every day counted with Trey. The doctors couldn't do the two tests on the same day. Postponing both until the following week would cause Trey to lose a precious day of some kind of treatment. It was a stall he couldn't afford.

We all knew it. It was hard to think, accept, and say out loud—but we all knew it. My resolve collapsed. For such a long time, I had kept the faith and entertained only positive thoughts and goals, making every environment as encouraging as it could be, surrounding myself with people who supported my high hopes. I had trusted Trey's needs to the prayer warriors who promised to follow through with petitions to God on his behalf. Through long searches for options, I never wavered from my and Charlie's vow to leave no stone unturned in the quest to save our son. Each time we stepped into a new arena of treatment, the hope was that this was where all those prayers and good thoughts had brought us.

All of that—and here we were. Intellectually, I always knew that melanoma had the power to take Trey, but in my heart, I never allowed myself to believe it would. More than ever, though, it now seemed to be bullying us.

This latest blow was a tough one, more than the kind that knocks the wind out of your sails. It shatters you from the inside out, bursting hearts and crushing spirits, unleashing your greatest fears and depleting your highest hopes. We'd had enough. We had just had enough, and after three years of trying to be the iron horse of strength and positivity, I finally crumbled. Oh, I had cried many times during our fight with melanoma, but this time I felt so defeated.

" . . . Now I'm falling apart . . . can't stop crying . . . " I typed in an email I sent to our family on May 13. Mainly, I was very concerned about Trey, because the news had been so much for him to take. Unable to stand the thought of him sitting around our Houston apartment during the worrisome weekend between spinal tests, I whisked us home on a six a.m. Saturday morning flight. We would have to return late Sunday night, but neither of us cared about the quick trip. Home was the only reprieve that could make the days ahead seem doable.

Trey

A lot of teenagers never want to hang around the house, but I've always liked being at home. When Mom booked the one-day trip from Houston to Atlanta and back again, I was glad to go. I loved the apartment in Houston. The Wade family made us feel so welcome, and I would never want to stay anywhere else, but . . . just not that weekend. I needed out of there just to clear my head.

The discovery of five new spots in my brain was a hard hit. Finding out the cancer might have made it to my brain and spinal fluid was even more devastating. I didn't think God was going to let me have more than I could handle, but, man, that felt like we were getting close to the limit.

I don't think I looked at the news the way a lot of people did, though. Considering the statistics on my disease, I guess there were people who thought I was getting into the final months of my life, but that wasn't where my mind was. Even though this was a huge wallop of bad news, I still believed it was just a setback. I would get well, but now I was really wondering just how many hurdles there were going to be before I finally got melanoma behind me. The most immediate worry was whether this latest news was going to keep me away from my high school graduation. Even if I was able to go to the ceremony, what was going to happen to my last summer on the lake before college? Would I even be able to start college on time? I hoped I wouldn't have to miss fraternity rush and move-in day at the dorms, as well as the UGA football games. I was still all about being a normal teenager, but instead of thinking like a high school student, I was thinking more and more about having a typical college life.

One hope I had that weekend between spinal tests was that the doctors only thought the melanoma might be in my brain and spinal fluid. They already had a plan in place in case the tests came back negative. I would go through ten days of low-dose brain radiation, which they said I could do in Atlanta. That was an awesome plan, and I tried to believe it would be the one we got. If the tests came back positive, my doctors would come up with another route. They didn't know what it would be, so maybe that was a good sign that it wouldn't be necessary anyway.

As things turned out, luck was on my side. On May 19, both the spinal MRI and spinal tap came back negative. There was no melanoma in my spine. It was a relief, to say the least. The doctors also decided not to do the brain radiation in Atlanta. Instead, I once again put on the Transformers-like headgear from my first gamma knife radiation to undergo a new one at MD Anderson. The doctors also harvested the surface tumors in my shoulder and ribs, to see if they could grow T-cells just in case I ended up needing them for a different trial. After that, I had two-and-a-half weeks off to go home and graduate. That's exactly what I was planning to do anyway.

Charlie

When Cherie and Trey got home from Houston, there was a lot to talk about. One of the topics was crawfish, and how many we would need for the big graduation party/crawfish boil we were hosting with five other families whose kids were also graduating from West Forsyth. Samantha Smith, Cailin Mace, Austin Todd, Nathan Teter, and Joey Moran had been friends of Trey's since their early years in elementary school. We held the party the Sunday before their Tuesday graduation. Putting it together was a big undertaking, with a final count of five hundred pounds of crawfish ordered. The fathers

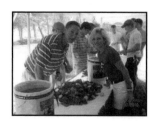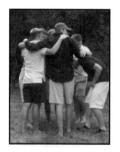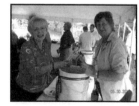

Trey with family and friends, graduation party at crawfish boil.

boiled and served them the traditional way—tossing them straight from buckets onto a long table covered in white paper, making for a true mess of crawdaddies, as they're often called. Some guests used plates, while others converged on the table to peel and eat while standing. My sons were in the latter group. It was a fun, laid-back afternoon. Even though there was some rainy weather in the area, we were set up under a big white tent in the Smiths' backyard.

This was exactly the kind of celebration Trey had most wanted. As he talked to guests, played volleyball, and dove for crawfish, he looked as much the part of a normal teenager as any of his friends did that day. His high school years had been far from normal, though. Cherie and I had tried to create as much normalcy around him as we could, while still prioritizing his health and treatments. We had to make a lot of decisions that aren't typical for a family with teenage sons, but Trey had his ways of letting us know that he thought we were doing the right thing. During his senior year, he gave us this handwritten note:

Dear Mom and Dad,

I have come a long way from when I first started playing football. Dad, you were my coach for years in different sports. Mom, you were always on the sideline with camera and yelling. If I could find the words to say or the things to do to thank you, I would say them or do whatever it is. I know sometimes it may not seem like it, but I love you both so much and you have always been there for me no matter what. Unfortunately, cancer has tried to get in the way of my high school career, but y'all were there to tell me I could do anything I put my mind to, and I have. My confidence and perseverance to beat this disease comes from both of you. I want to thank you again for always being there for me and just know that I will always love you no matter what.

Love, Trey

Cherie

For Charlie and me, just considering the possibility that we would be home for Trey's graduation to watch him walk across the stage was a huge blessing all by itself.

After the gamma knife radiation on Trey's five new brain tumors, we would have to wait three weeks to see if any new tumors had shown up. If not, he should be eligible to begin the ipilimumab drug trial. The problem was that time wasn't on our side if Trey ended up not being a candidate for the trial. Subcutaneous tumors had begun showing up almost daily all over his body. For the first time, he could even feel one of the tumors on his shoulder. It was painfully, terrifyingly obvious that Trey's cancer was progressing faster than it ever had before.

We had to be prepared to immediately move on to something different if the clinical trial was taken off the table. We talked through many options with Dr. Hwu and Trey, going through so many possibilities and information overload. We had been reading and talking with other patients. I had stayed on blogs in a quest to become as educated as possible about most of the options. We kind of had plans A, B, C, and D in our heads or written in our notes, but the more we researched, the more we went far beyond all those thoughts. It was completely overwhelming and frustrating to have so much information, with no answer, no plan should we need it.

Then came the idea from Dr. Hwu to go ahead and harvest or resect three of Trey's pea- and lima bean-size subcutaneous tumors and see if they would grow T-cells. One immediate hurdle was that there wasn't an operating room available to get the tumors resected in time to get Trey home for graduation. This news was devastating to Trey, who had been so close to making that goal of walking with his class.

Dr. Hwu's other idea was to perform the resection in a clinic room, as long as a surgeon was available and a lab tech was waiting to immediately take the cells to the lab. It was underway the very next day, with Charlie and me actually sitting on a bench in the corner of the room, watching the process, and talking to the surgeon through it all. Trey was conscious. All the doctors had to do was apply a topical numbing agent to the areas where they were removing each tumor by needle injection, so it wasn't too painful an ordeal for Trey. Our conversation and observation were made comfortable, but our nerves were fraying. Hope was so high, but there was much anxiety centered on nothing going wrong so that this could be Trey's answer.

Since we weren't in a normal operating room, Dr. Hwu had arranged for a lab technician to be present, quietly waiting behind the curtained entrance area of the room. After each tumor was precisely cut out and carefully placed in a small laboratory tube, they were immediately handed to the technician, who safely transported them to the lab where every attempt would be made to encourage T-cell growth. What we didn't know until much later was that the lab technician made a detour to the pathology department, where the tumors were treated to preserve them. Without that stop, they wouldn't have been good to grow the T-cells everyone wanted to see.

After the resection, Trey was stitched up. Then we were on our way back to Atlanta for graduation, knowing that all we could do was take one day at a time and stay positive. Trying to make the best out of each and every day, I stayed focused on what was coming up and that was graduation. I had prepared for the graduation party as much as I could in between trips to Houston, and with the help of other parents. We wanted Trey and his friends to have the best graduation party we could give them.

All of our family came to town for graduation. It was so big to all of us that we had reached this point. After all, we could never be sure if we would see this day. It was kind of surreal when people asked me how Trey was doing and we'd tell them he'd already fought off nine brain tumors since February, and how we were hoping there wouldn't be any more before Trey's clinical trial started in June. We were also praying hard that Trey's cells were growing, since they might become our only good option. We had already adjusted to so many game changes that we were now ready to take on any new plan at any given moment.

For the time being, however, the focus was on one thing: Trey was home for graduation. The crawfish boil graduation party was a hit, resulting in a priceless smile on Trey's face as he joined in the fun with all of his friends, living life like a normal high-school-graduate-turned-college-student. That smile was a gift to Charlie and me. I was devoted in my resolve to see this trial as a positive, a solution, not something to dread. Though I had suffered a huge meltdown and crying jag earlier in May, I rallied quickly and was back to my positivity stance. I absolutely could not, would not, tolerate any negativity from anyone or anything. No matter how grave things may have appeared to most, I challenged myself to seek out the good. Whenever people asked me about Trey, and every time I wrote an update, I sought the silver lining and tried to make others see and feel my belief that Trey was going to win this, somehow, some way, some day.

We were tremendously proud that Trey would be going to the University of Georgia, but it was hard to even think about it right then. In between that and the graduation was another trip to Houston, and whatever followed. August 9 was his freshman move-in date at UGA, but it was ten weeks away, and seemed so far into the future against our present reality. I knew summer would pass quickly, but we just had to put that date on the backburner. It was very hard to look too far into the future, since we could barely even plan out one week that might not see a sudden change in the game plan.

The day of graduation, surrounded by our family, was so incredible that I almost had to pinch myself for assurance that it was all for real. Sometimes I just could not believe we had actually made it that far. Trey had barely been able to make it to school for a lot of his senior year, but there we were, watching him walk across the stage to get his high school diploma. Against high medical odds, Charlie and I were among all the other parents—cheering, applauding, and beaming—looking as if nothing had ever happened.

Trey

On June 1, 2010, I walked across the stage to get my high school diploma. It's a milestone for everyone, but it really felt like a huge personal one to me considering how up and down the past few years had been.

There were over four hundred people in my class, so graduation was held at the Gwinnett Civic Center in Duluth. Each time someone was handed their diploma, their name and any honors flashed across the large screen on the back wall of the stage. When it was my turn to cross, the screen read:

Trey Rood
Honor Graduate
Rotary Scholarship
$2500

I had just found out a few weeks earlier about the scholarship from the Rotary Club of Forsyth County. The actual name was the "2010 Challenge Scholarship" and the school counselors nominated the students who received it. For me, that was my counselor, Mr. Carnaroli, who had worked to keep me on track toward graduation.

Afterward, a ton of pictures were taken of me and my friends, mostly by our parents. We went back a lot of years together, but this day was a symbol of the changing directions we would all be heading toward. Everybody had their plans. My plans were to go back to Houston for whatever awaited me there. After that, I was going to the University of Georgia in Athens. I wasn't sure when I would get there, or what I'd go through to get there, but I knew I would get there.

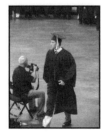

Trey attends high school graduation on June 1, 2010.

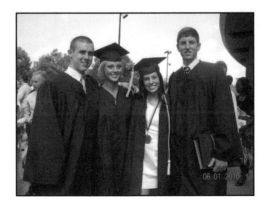

Chapter Sixteen

Cherie

High school graduation is supposed to mark new beginnings. Charlie and I could only hope that meant new beginnings for Trey as we got ready to return with him to MD Anderson in June. He was scheduled to start the trial on June 11. This had to be the one that would turn things around.

Wes appeared to be hanging in there. His grandmother was staying with him most of the time while we were gone, but since he hadn't made any trips to Houston, I often wondered what he imagined was happening. I knew in my heart that family and friends took good care of Wes, and I prayed daily that he would understand and be okay with not having parents around as much as we wanted to be. I couldn't let myself get too worried about it, because there was no alternative. We had to do what we could to save Trey. Hopefully the end result would be many, many more years together as a family of four, and plenty of opportunities for our sons to enjoy life together.

Before heading back to MD Anderson, we felt guided by the biblical instructions of James 5:14: "Is any among you sick? Let him call for the elders of the church, and let them pray over him, anointing him with oil in the name of the Lord." The urge to follow this was so strong that we knew we couldn't board a plane to Houston without first meeting with ministers from Browns Bridge Community Church. With Kevin Ragsdale's assistance, on the very day we were to fly out, Pastor Lane Brown anointed Trey with oil, laid hands on him, and prayed with us that God would restore Trey's body with complete healing. Only when that was done did we feel blessed with the strength needed to continue on the journey forced upon us by melanoma.

We would need it right away, because on June 10, another new spot had appeared on the MRI for Trey's brain. The spot was tiny, which was good, but it was new and thus delayed the clinical trial again. Another gamma knife treatment was scheduled to knock this additional brain tumor out, Trey's fourth time under gamma.

We were, however, very encouraged to learn that the tumor tissue harvested for T-cell therapy had grown! It had actually grown very well. The process for starting Trey in a T-cell trial was immediately under way. Once again, the closing of one door was followed by the opening of another. This one led to a detailed process, which included five days of harsh chemotherapy, T-cell infusion, and more rounds of IL-2. It was also possible that Trey would be a candidate for the randomized selection process to receive a boost of dendritic cells to help direct the T-cells to attack the cancer. It would be a long and hard road for Trey, but a one-time process. So far, results showed that it had a better response rate than the original trial Trey was being tested for. A possible bonus was that it also showed the ability to fight off brain tumors in many cases.

The doctors' honesty about how difficult treatment would be was met with dread and trepidation about how Trey's summer would go. It crippled any good feelings about the process. The doctors, though, had not expected to see his T-cells grow as they had. The fact that they did was huge. This was our green light to move forward. The trial would require a three-week stay at MD Anderson in early July. There would be follow up with another week in the hospital after that, and that was the extent of treatment.

It took what seemed like forever to find out if Trey had been chosen through the randomized selection process to receive dendritic cells. I remember pushing so hard for this with the research nurse at the time. I wanted every assurance we were throwing everything in that we could to maybe, just maybe, help this T-cell treatment be successful.

A couple weeks before treatment was scheduled to begin, we returned home to make the best of whatever we could of any summer fun with family and friends. It actually turned out to be a very good time, starting with Trey being awarded "AJC Inspirational Athlete of the Year" from the

Atlanta Journal-Constitution on June 13. They wrote a moving article that paid tribute to his positive attitude. West Forsyth Coach David Rooney, one of Trey's mentors, said:

I've seen him after he's lost 20 pounds out there on the field and had to take extra water breaks. Then I'd turn around and he'd be next to me saying "Coach, I'm ready to go back in." Other times, I've seen him when he felt absolutely great and been a leader to everyone out there.

Trey's friend and teammate Nathan Teter was quoted saying:

I think it's unbelievable. I just don't see how someone at his young age, struck down with news like that, can keep going with such a wonderful attitude. He always stays motivated and never gives up on anything. I think that is what has really helped him out with his treatments. He is always pushing and trying in everything he does."

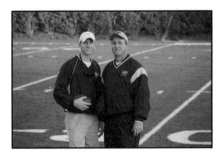

Trey with mentor and coach, David Rooney.

Another thing we were talking about was Trey's plans for college. Maybe some people thought we were over-the-top unrealistic, but I decided to start thinking of move-in day the same way Trey was—he would be among thousands of other students arriving on campus that day. I joined some girlfriends on a college shopping trip. We each loaded up our respective rising freshman with dorm décor, linens, and everything else they might need to start their new lives.

Trey and I attended Freshman Orientation, where he registered for classes scheduled to begin on August 16. It was either a step of faith, or we were completely crazy, but we trusted this whole thing was going to time out perfectly for Trey, just like so many other things had. While we were there, Trey also signed up for fraternity rush, had his student identification card made, and selected his meal plan.

On one of our recent trips to Houston, Trey had cognitive testing done for memory loss due to the radiation, gamma knife, and brain surgery. Short-term memory loss was going to be an issue. Knowing this helped us get him signed up with the UGA Disability Resource Center (DRC) and assigned to a case manager. The DRC provided Trey more time for test and note taking, in addition to early-access class registration. Not knowing how long he would need help, we made sure he had it if he would benefit from it. I felt the DRC could build Trey's confidence, since he was jumping back into school after having missed a lot during his senior year of high school.

I had my worries and, like many mothers, one of them was Trey's living arrangements once he got to UGA. I knew he would be settling into a dorm, but we didn't know who his roommate would be, since it was all lottery-based. I really wished he was living with a friend, someone who knew what he had been through and might be quick to notice any subtle changes that could indicate a health problem.

While we were in Athens making all the college preparations, we found out that our friend and next door neighbor Austin Todd had made some changes in his college plans. Though he'd planned to attend Wake Forest University, he decided to stay closer to home and attend UGA instead. I talked to his mom Dee, running the possibility of Trey and Austin rooming together by her. We quickly agreed that this would be great for both of them, but weren't quite sure how to make it happen. With fall semester starting in less than two months, the deadline for requesting a specific roommate had closed well before our idea came together.

Everything changed the minute I lamented our conundrum to my friend Lisa Slocum, who lives in Athens. Unbeknownst to me, she was well acquainted with Rodney Bennett, UGA's dean of student affairs, and quickly arranged a meeting between us. By "quickly," I mean I was walking into his office twenty minutes after she made a phone call to him! During that meeting, I barely got my concerns out on the table when he said, "Check that off your list." Not only was I assured that Trey and Austin would room together, but they were placed in what he promised was the best room in Oglethorpe House, a nine-story dormitory with bedroom suites. Their new digs included a semi-private bath. The building was connected to one of the four campus dining halls. I wasn't sure what needs Trey would have after T-cell therapy. After all, we were still living one day at a time. By trying to plan ahead and stay positive, he would get to move into his dorm with Austin as we hoped. The timing was another one of those God-things, and Mr. Bennett was another one of our angels. While I left feeling very good about things, there was one comment Mr. Bennett made during our meeting that stayed with me. He said that if Trey had to miss up to two weeks at the beginning of the semester, he would need to withdraw. We just couldn't let that happen.

Before we returned to Houston, Trey got invited to a summer rush party hosted by Sigma Chi fraternity. Not only was Trey a legacy to Sigma Chi, but a bid to pledge would make him a fourth-generation Sigma Chi in the Delta chapter at UGA. I don't know much about the party he attended, but assume he had a great time since he wound up spending the entire weekend with the guys!

On July 6, Trey and I again took our seats on another Atlanta-to-Houston flight. He arrived in Houston with one thing already checked off the long list of things he would be put through: getting a PICC (peripherally inserted central catheter) line placed into his chest at Scottish-Rite Children's Hospital in Atlanta. We took any chance we had to get something done on our own home turf. Getting his line placement in exchange for an extra day at home was worth it.

As things got under way, Trey's attitude remained on top of the game plan, never seeming to waver, fueled by his faith and the messages from friends back home. I often heard him talking on the phone. While I could only catch his side of the conversation, I knew the calls were from UGA fraternity guys inviting him to more summer rush events. It saddened me to hear him decline, but he'd never tell them why.

Treatment was delayed by one day. After arriving at the hospital and getting settled into the room, we learned that Trey's T-cells needed to thaw out. The staff needed to confirm that the one hundred billion T-cells extracted from his tumors had grown. For Trey, any delay was too long, so this unexpected news wasn't welcome. But we were elated to find out they were thriving and Trey could begin chemotherapy. Unlike many treatments where chemo is used to attack cancer cells, it would have a different role in T-cell therapy: it would be used to deplete Trey's body of most lymphocytes, to make room for the T-cells and dendritic cells he would receive.

Almost every day during chemo week, with IV pole in tow, I walked Trey to the Oaks, a restaurant inside Rotary House International Hotel on the MD Anderson campus. As long as his appetite was up for it, Trey was happy to be treated to a good steak dinner and enjoy a change of scenery. The Wades usually met up with us—and with Charlie in Atlanta for Wes, it was especially comforting to me to have their companionship. This was just another way the Wade family blessed us being so far away from home. They were so incredibly compassionate.

Even though the three-week hospital stay felt like a long cut into Trey's summer, every day brought something new. It might have been starting a different part of treatment, enjoying quality time with the Wades, watching the World Cup Soccer Tournament, or shopping online for dorm room items.

Trey endured the chemo pretty well and was ready to begin the infusions of T-cells and dendritic cells. I will never forget the day this part of treatment began. Trey seemed to be on center stage as a small and cloudy white bag of fluid was carefully brought in and connected to his IV. It was like the bag was filled with pure liquid gold, a precious treasure that demanded the most secure, delicate attention and care. The truth was, it was precious, because it held the hope of life for Trey.

Next came a blizzard of "white coats"—doctors filing in and out of the room and nurses lining the walls—all there to witness a remarkable, historic event as an eighteen-year-old became one of the first people in the world to receive this infusion combination and have this done on the melanoma floor of MD Anderson. Many treatments of this sort were instead performed in ICU. I gazed about the room in awe, realizing just how monumental this really was. This was groundbreaking research even at a huge, established hospital like MD Anderson. The scene around me was almost dreamlike as I turned my eyes to Trey, waiting in his hospital bed for what he trusted was a "miracle-in-a-bag" God had delivered. The name of my own flesh and blood would be forever written in the pages of medical history. The enormity of that thought was knee-buckling. I was sorry we needed to be there, yet so grateful, and I was proud—proud of Trey, and every person in that room for the hope they might give other patients with this cancer diagnosis.

The T-cells traveled through Trey's IV over the course of twenty minutes. Under the watchful eyes of doctors, he had some of the expected side effects, chills, shaking, and nausea, from which he recovered after about four hours. Then it was time for the infusion of dendritic cells, which had been spun (or made) from Trey's own blood.

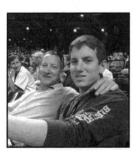

June 2010, Charlie and Trey caught a Houston Astros game, compliments of Roger Clemens.

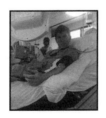

Trey's summer treatments (in 2010) started with him having hair.

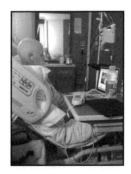

By the end of treatments, Trey lost his hair.

Thankfully, Trey didn't show too many side effects from the dendritic cells infusion. The worst of those effects came during the dreaded IL-2 treatments, which followed the infusions and completed the full program of T-cell therapy. Trey's two previous rounds of IL-2 had been documented for the kinds of side effects doctors might expect for him, so everyone was on high alert in an attempt to stay ahead of them. The biggest concern from Trey's IL-2 history was that his heart rate always sped off the charts, forcing doctors to stop the treatment. To try to avoid it this time, he was placed on the beta-blocker Toprol. His heart still outran the medication. This caused some major difficulties when he was several doses into our early-August second round of IL-2 to complete the entire T-cell therapy treatment. Panicked, he shot up in bed one night feeling like he couldn't breathe, swallow, or move in any capacity. His heart rate scared us both. Doctors and nurses stormed the room with no time to waste. Just as they were about to rush him to ICU, Trey's heart returned to a normal and regular pumping cycle.

After that frightening episode, Trey understandably decided that enough was enough. Usually so mild and compliant with whatever it took, this time he firmly announced, "I'm done. I can't take this anymore. No more rounds of IL-2."

Though I expected the treatments to resume, Trey's doctors actually did agree that he'd had enough, not only mentally and physically, but also enough for the T-cell therapy to be successful. While I hoped that was true, what if stopping the IL-2 early impacted the outcome negatively?

Trey

It only took five days of chemo before my hair started falling out. There's a difference in choosing to have your head shaved clean and watching your hair come out on its own, leaving nothing but wisps behind. Up until then, and through all the melanoma treatments, I hadn't ever really looked sick. Now I was starting to look like the cancer patient I was, and I worried some about what people thought when they saw me. I checked the mirror every day to see how much more bald I'd gotten since the day before.

For whatever reason, God didn't want me on the clinical trial originally planned. I just accepted that this new one was going to be better. Mom called it one of the "granddaddies" of medical research, and a historical point in the road we'd traveled. We were all pumped that the harvested T-cells from a few of my surface tumors had grown so well, and that we could use them to fight and kill all of my tumors. I'd developed a lot of new tumors lately. It seemed like every couple of days I was showing one to Mom.

Overall, the chemo really wasn't so bad. Losing my hair was the biggest side effect. Boredom was my largest hurdle, as I just waited to get out of the hospital to preserve what was left of the summer. I wanted to get in some golf and wakeboarding before moving to Athens for school, and attending some of the fraternity rush events I'd been invited to.

The T-cell and dendritic cell infusions also went pretty smoothly, but when the IL-2 treatments came along, the doctors said they were giving me all the IL-2 that I could take. They weren't kidding. It was tough, with the heart episode being one of the scariest things to happen in the whole scope of dealing with melanoma. My heart was pounding so hard that I could hear it in my head. It really felt like it was going to rip and explode right through my chest. My throat and lungs felt full of cement—hardening by the second. I really don't know what went through my mind during the actual episode, but I know what I was thinking when it ended: it was time to stop IL-2. It would just be a short break, though. I already knew that when the T-cell therapy was over with, I'd have a week off before returning again for another dose of IL-2, which would be the first week in August. If all went well, I would be able to make my planned move-in date of August 10 at my freshman dorm at UGA. I couldn't wait for the day when I'd never have to hear that term again: IL-2.

After the whole T-cell therapy treatment and first round of IL-2, I left the hospital in late July weighing twenty pounds less than I had when I arrived. That would have been a real concern back when I was playing football. Now it just made me more self-conscious about what I looked like, more than anything—if people automatically thought "he's sick with something" when they looked at me. I still just wanted to be normal.

We hadn't been home in Atlanta long when I got another invitation to hang out with some Sigma Chi brothers from UGA. They were going to an Atlanta Braves game at Turner Field, close to home. The first time I'd met these guys, I had hair. Now I was bald, but at least we were going to a baseball game where ball caps were the norm!

There were other guys there who were also rushing. None of them looked at me strangely or anything, but when I told one of the guys, Wills Aitkens, my name, his eyes grew big.

"No way!" he said. That kind of threw me. "Man, you're a legend!"

Turns out, Wills had attended Holy Innocents, a private school in the Atlanta area. Wills and his football coach had the whole team pray for me. The coach had even given the entire football team "Pray for Trey" wristbands to wear.

I was always amazed to meet a stranger—someone I didn't know, but who knew all about me and had been praying for me. I'd never been called a "legend" before, though. It didn't fit the way I saw myself at all! Right then, I was just a guy hoping to get a bid to pledge Sigma Chi.

Charlie

Cherie and I helped move Trey into the dorms at UGA. After the last IL-2 treatment in early August, we barely made his move-in date of August 10. We flew back to Atlanta on a Monday night, and move-in started Tuesday morning. There was Trey, ready to start college and pledge Sigma Chi. The bid he wanted had been offered and he would be joining the same chapter in the same house I had pledged years earlier.

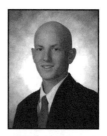

Trey's first official Sigma Chi photo.

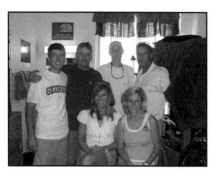

Move-in day on the UGA campus with the Todd family.

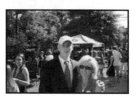

Trey and Cherie tailgating at the Sigma Chi house.

He hadn't been at UGA long before it was time for another follow up at MD Anderson on August 24, where he'd undergo scans to check his response to the T-cell therapy. A week before returning, he was already noticing that some surface tumors were gone, smaller or less painful. We took it as a good sign.

We'd endured a few hard blows on these follow-up visits, but this one showed that the primary tumor in Trey's lung had shrunk considerably along with many others. This was phenomenal news we'd waited so long to hear.

However, there was a bit of cold water thrown on our good news when they discovered another tumor had appeared—this time on the pelvis bone. Dr. Hwu wasn't worried, though, saying the tumor was really small and that those in the bone were the last to respond to T-cell therapy. The brain MRI also showed another new spot that was bleeding out. Again, Dr. Hwu wasn't overly concerned about it, because it was so small in size and would undergo another treatment with gamma knife radiation. Overall, Dr. Hwu felt positive. We all agreed with Cherie, who said, "Today is still a good day!"

Trey quickly immersed himself in his new life at UGA. We were fortunate to get to enjoy a lot of it with him: going to Athens for football games and pre-game tailgates at the Sigma Chi house, packed with active brothers and pledges, dates, alums, and parents spilling out onto the front lawn for live music and food. Cherie quickly got involved with the Sigma Chi Mothers' Club. Life felt as good as it could during those stretches between visits to MD Anderson. Most of our friends with new college freshman students talked so much about how they were having a hard time with their son or daughter leaving home to start college, and how much they were missing them. Cherie and I never had those thoughts. We were so happy Trey was actually in college, that he had made it this far! It was wonderful watching him enjoying life, behaving and living like the normal college kid he wanted so badly to be.

We had to yank Trey away from his new life a lot to make those return visits, but he never really complained. They were intrusive, sure, but his attitude was more of a "let's get this over with" approach so he could hurry back to his world at UGA. Happily, as time went on, those visits were spread out over longer spans of time.

Trey

In the middle of September, halfway through my Sigma Chi pledgeship, I returned to Houston to take care of one final brain tumor. This was the little tumor that had shown up on my more recent brain MRI in late August.

Just Mom and I made the trip to Houston, which marked the fifth time in about six months that I would strap on the headgear and go through a long day of gamma knife radiation. The light at the end of the tunnel was that after radiation, we'd take a trip to see my friend Cailin, who was now a freshman at Florida State University in Tallahassee. Mom had rented a car for the trip, which meant I'd get to leave Houston quicker than usual. The doctors forbade me from flying for twenty-four to forty-eight hours after gamma knife. Traveling in a car was fine right after the treatment, though.

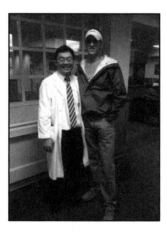

Dr. Patrick Hwu and Trey pose at MD Anderson after first positive test results following T-cell therapy.

Cailin's mom Dodi flew down to Houston to join us for the drive to Tallahassee. Cailin was in her first busy season on one of FSU's football cheerleading squads. At some point during all the long-distance talking and hanging out during my short trips home, she and I had started dating, so I was really looking forward to seeing her. I did some of the driving too. It was so good to be out of the hospital. The open road felt great, like I was on a new path to freedom. It was a ten-hour drive, but nothing we couldn't handle. We had a great weekend in Tallahassee visiting with Cailin, but it was soon time to return home—which meant back to UGA and the Sigma Chi life for me.

Charlie

The updates that went on the web and social media pages were a testament to the answered prayers and to the great work done by Dr. Patrick Hwu and his team at MD Anderson.

Great News From Houston
10-6-2010

Trey returned to Houston on Monday for more scans and MRIs. We got the best report in quite some time: ALL tumors are shrinking! Nor are there any new tumors. Trey will return to Houston in six weeks for more scans. Please pray for continued improvement. Thanks so much for all your support and continued prayers. Go God!

What a Great Start to the New Year!
1-5-2011

Trey's appointment today in Houston could not have gone better. His brain is still clear, his tumors continue to shrink, and no new tumors were discovered anywhere. His doctor took Trey off all medications and he doesn't have to come back again for three months. We are so excited. God is good! Thank you for all of your awesome prayers.

Awesome News
3-30-2011

All of Trey's CT scans came back stable. There's nothing new and the brain MRI remains clear. There are several tumors we continue to watch.

As it stands now, they are either smaller in size or are not getting any larger (stable). Additionally, there is no way to tell from the scans if they are live tumors or dead tumors absorbing slowly into his body (calcification/scar tissue showing up). The only way to know for sure is to surgically remove and test each tumor, which is not an option at this point. Why crack his chest open and remove a lung to see if a stable or shrinking tumor has live cancer cells or not?

Dr. Hwu said he would be happy for everything to stay stable as it is for the next 60 years. We'll take it! We want to keep Trey healthy and his stress level low, but at the same time enjoy life and be as normal as possible. As many of you know, all his hair has grown back. It's a little too curly for his liking, but a small thing in the big picture. He doesn't need to be back at MD Anderson for another four months (end of July). He is so excited to have a summer this year. Praise God. It's a great day. "PFT"

Heading Back to Houston
8-8-2011

We can't say enough to thank everyone for your support and continued prayers for Trey. It's that time again. We are heading back to Houston today for Trey to go through all the usual CT scans, MRIs, and doctor appointments. Trey has been doing great and living life as a typical college student in Athens at the University of Georgia. It's just so good to see him have the freedom and time to enjoy life. Need we say more?

It's been just over a year (July 2010) since Trey underwent "Adoptive T-cell Therapy" at MD Anderson. We have seen incredible results. It has stabilized his stage IV melanoma. In March, some tumors were no longer there, while others were stable or not growing. The biggest success was that nothing new had shown up, particularly in his brain. For this reason, we want to ask for your continued prayers for continued success and complete healing as we return to Houston this week.

We are so blessed and grateful for the miracle that he is. Prayer is awesome! Thank you and God Bless. Keeping the faith. Go God!

More Encouraging News
8-10-2011

We got great news for Trey today. He doesn't have any new tumors. His brain is still clear. And all other tumor areas remain stable—if not smaller. Trey gets another 4 months off before coming back to MD Anderson for the same scans, MRIs, and doctor appointments again. We are so incredibly blessed!

Trey's oncologist, Dr. Patrick Hwu, is using Trey's story to encourage other patients. He wanted Trey to know how many people he is inspiring and that his recovery is giving hope to others. He wanted to encourage Trey to continue to live life to the fullest. God is working miracles through Trey. Go God!

Trey's New Scans are Encouraging
12-14-2011

Trey's brain MRI and CT scans "could not have been better," to quote his oncologist, Dr. Patrick Hwu. His brain was clear and scans showed smaller tumors and potentially dead tissue. His doctor gave Trey five months off before coming back to do this all over again. What a true blessing and miracle Trey continues to be.

Thank you for all your prayers. Go God!

Trey Is Our Miracle Again!
05-09-2012

Trey's brain MRI was clear and all CT scans were good. His doctor said he's doing the best that they could expect. We're so excited for Trey. He'll start his summer college courses tomorrow morning!

Go God! Thank you for all your prayers.

Heading Back for Tests
08-06-2012

It's that time again. We are headed back to Houston with Trey this Tuesday and Wednesday for his scheduled CT scans, brain MRI, and doctor appointments. It has only been three months since Trey had his last round of tests. He starts his junior year at UGA next week and didn't want to return to MD Anderson in the middle of fall semester. The doctors agreed to see him earlier so he wouldn't have to come back again until right after the holidays. Trey is now exactly two years out of T-cell treatment. What a miracle he is! Please pray for continued response and great test results this week. Go God!

Great Results!
08-12-2012

Trey's test results were great—clear of tumors and nothing new. Trey doesn't have to come back to do this all over again until December 18th! MD Anderson actually filmed Trey from a patient's perspective for their website on T-cell therapy. It is very cool to see how Trey's story is inspiring other patients and giving them hope.

Praise God!

Praise God!
12-19-2012

Trey's test results were good. There was nothing new. He was released for six months before we have to come back to MD Anderson to do this all over again!

Trey continues to be our miracle. Praise God!

Those updates were a long way from the earlier ones we posted that were sometimes grim and, at best, only cautiously optimistic. I don't know if anyone was surprised to see Trey's incredible progress against melanoma, but I know someone who wasn't surprised—and that was Trey. He always expected it and his only real question was "How long until I get there?"

Chapter Seventeen

Trey

In between my trips to Houston, there has been a lot of living. Going to class, studying, fraternity meetings, sporting events, hanging out—a lot of things that make up a normal college life. I think about melanoma when it's time to go to Houston for scans, but only as something I have to check up on. I'm not fighting off worry that it might come back, or wondering what happens if it ever does. God has a plan, and I'm good with that. I felt that way even during the darkest times, so I'm not about to be stressing now that I believe melanoma is behind me.

People continue to support me in every way, but one of the biggest groups to surround me in recent years is my fraternity. I love Sigma Chi. I love everything it was founded on and what it means to me now. None of these guys knew me when the whole melanoma fight started, but they've supported me like they were there from day one. One of the best things they did was kick off an event in the spring of 2011 called "Trey Rood Band of Brothers." This incorporated a number of fundraisers, with the goal of raising fifty thousand dollars by the end of the year for Dr. Hwu's melanoma research at MD Anderson. That was really cool.

Two of my now closest friends are pledge brothers, Ryan Holden and Chris Kasuya. Their impression of me and melanoma is similar to the views of my high school friends. I hope that shows I've been consistent in my attitude and, mainly, in my faith.

Ryan Holden

I'm from Pittsburgh, Pennsylvania, and when I first got to UGA and started fraternity rush, it seemed like all I saw were guys in Polo shirts and sunglasses. For someone like me, who looks like he's stepped right out of the TV show Jersey Shore, this was culture shock.

The first time I met Trey was when he picked me up for our first pledge class meeting. It was the Sunday night before classes started. I was standing outside my dorm when Trey roared up in his truck. We have trucks in Pittsburgh, but nothing like the ones these southern boys drive. Trey's was a silver Toyota Tundra, lifted with loud pipes and nicknamed "the grey hound."

Wow, I thought, as it stopped in front of me. What in the hell is that? I climbed inside the cab with Trey and could tell right away that he was really tall—and that he had no hair. I didn't immediately think of cancer, but instead wondered if maybe he had an autoimmune disease or something like that. Whatever was going on with him, he was friendly and confident. Once we got to the meeting, he really seemed to be having a great time with everyone. It was at this meeting that Trey told everyone he had cancer.

My dad, also a Sigma Chi from the UGA Delta chapter, once had Hodgkin's disease. He's fine now, but I remember when he was going through it, and how stressful it can be for someone dealing with treatment and side effects. After the meeting, I went to Trey and offered to talk if he ever wanted to.

Even though I'd go on to find out that cancer is something Trey rarely talks about, the subject of illness was a commonality we had, so maybe that was our initial connection. We quickly learned, though, that we were polar opposites. For example, Trey loves the outdoors and was into hunting and fishing. I had never been on a boat, let alone hunted or fished.

It took a little while, but we discovered that we got a kick out of each other's differences and grew comfortable giving each other crap about them—like him calling me a "northern guido." This helped as we made our way through pledgeship, which can be hard and time-consuming. We had a great pledge group. There were thirty of us, and we were close-knit. Even though we're all initiated brothers now, we're still an inner circle where there is always someone to talk to and help carry hardships.

Trey amazed everyone during pledgeship. After what he'd been through all summer, and later with trips back and forth to Houston, I know he had to be exhausted some days. He never complained about the life of a pledge, always pulled his weight, was on time for meetings, and knew his fraternity history. If he was feeling anything negative about his cancer, nobody knew it, because he never wore his emotions on his sleeve.

Whenever anyone asked Trey how he was doing, or if pledging was getting to be too much, his answer was always the same: "I'm good." By the time pledgeship ended, Trey and I were close friends and I was really looking forward to some time to relax. Not Trey, though. The very day after pledging ended, Trey said he really wanted to get in shape.

"Let's take some time off," I suggested, "and just enjoy our free time."

Trey wasn't interested in that. "Look, I was a football player and can't be complacent," he told me. "Plus, I've been through hell, and I'm not gonna sit here and do nothing."

Before I knew it, he had me in the gym lifting weights with him six days a week. This went on during our entire second semester of school. Because he'd been sick, I was nervous in the beginning as to whether we should be training so much, but Trey proved he was able to handle it. Really, our lifting was pretty ugly for both of us at first, but we worked up to where we were neck and neck on how much weight we could each handle. After two months of being dead even, Trey broke loose and blew me out of the water. By that point, he had put weight back on and was so strong.

Another thing Trey wanted to work on was pre-calculus, which was a required course for both of us at UGA. Because Trey had missed a lot of lessons in high school, he was struggling with this math class. After working out at the gym, we'd head over to see a tutor. I knew Trey had some memory problems after the brain tumors, but it was incredible how he started excelling in that class. I was seeing more and more that Trey is never content. He always wanted to do better, to improve, to excel. For me, someone who had wanted some down time after pledging, Trey's drive was both inspiring and humbling.

Since they were a few years apart in age, my dad and Trey's dad didn't know each other too well during their undergrad years in Sigma Chi. Our parents are close now, and I feel like Trey and I have an inner-family thing also connecting us. Distance keeps me from getting home too often, but Trey's family always welcomes me to spend Easter or any other time with them.

Cancer having touched my family too, I understand what people go through watching a loved one deal with treatment. I respect what Trey has been through and I respect who he is. I think everyone in Sigma Chi does, as well, and I can say that his supporting cast at UGA is second to none. At a school with almost thirty-five thousand students, Trey is one person who is liked by everyone who gets a chance to meet him.

For me, though, the northern guy on a big southern campus where it's easy to get lost—Trey Rood has made the University of Georgia feel a whole lot smaller.

Chris Kasuya

Like Trey, I'm from Georgia, having gone to high school in Marietta, which isn't too far from Trey's hometown of Cumming. The first time I ever saw him was at the Saturday night party for new Sigma Chi pledges. I noticed he was bald, but really didn't think much about it. Instead, I asked someone, "Who's that guy?"

"That's Trey Rood," they told me. "He's a big-time legacy to this house."

Legacy or not, Trey just looked like a cool guy who seemed to be having a good time. I walked over to introduce myself and said, "Congrats on your bid. It looks like we're going to be pledge brothers."

At that moment, I didn't realize how very important Trey Rood would become to me, starting with our pledgeship the fall of our freshman year. The next night was our first pledge meeting, where we were asked to go around the room to introduce ourselves and share one "interesting fact" about ourselves. I don't imagine anyone will ever forget Trey's introduction.

"I'm Trey Rood—and I'm fighting cancer."

Pledging is tough, but Trey never held back, never did less than anyone else, and would go on to finish as one of the top ten pledges in our class. Watching him stay on top and always do his share, despite all he'd just gone through that summer, was humbling and impressive. I don't know if Trey realizes how much he impacted our pledge class to keep life in perspective. When guys would complain about the time and work of pledging, and say how bad their lives felt at the moment, someone would always bring up Trey. We all knew he'd been struggling through his life, and that he was still fighting to recover, yet he was the one who never complained. Without any words, and just by the way he went through his days, he was showing everyone that living and breathing are good and not to be taken for granted. He helped everyone keep it real by reminding us that the big picture was more important than any temporary thing happening at the moment.

I think there are three ways people can approach college life. They can spend all their time studying and not utilizing the years to grow and experience other parts of life; they can decide not to focus at all on academics and waste the main reason they go to school; or they can balance their academic, social, and other activities, and make the years well-rounded. Trey is definitely in the third category, plus he was having to balance it all with trips to and from MD Anderson. He was, and is, living a great example of my favorite quote: "Life is ten percent what happens to you and ninety percent how you deal with it."

During pledgeship, Trey and I spent a lot of time together while cleaning the Sigma Chi house. That is probably when our friendship really started to strengthen, because we always tried to turn the work into fun. Being around him drove home how much we all need to cherish the little things. We had plenty of opportunity to talk and covered a lot of ground. Cancer wasn't really one of them, though, because it's something Trey just didn't dwell on. He wasn't afraid to talk about it. Trey was never scared of that, but when he did talk, it seemed intentional. He wanted it to serve a purpose for whoever was listening. This went along with his trust in God, and believing that God would give him reasons to use his experience to help bless others.

Trey was accepted into UGA's Terry College of Business, majoring in finance. I'm studying international business and see myself traveling all over the world. This plan is different than the one Trey has in mind, because he's more of a homebody than I am. We both want to be successful and reach our destinations, but also think we can combine our strengths to one day start a company together.

Trey has also decided that he wants to get into public speaking. That's awesome—not only because it would be good for our future company, but also because Trey could step out and inspire others with the story of his battle against melanoma. I'm proud of him for that and think it's an important thing to do. He's never seen cancer as something that held him back. Even though it knocked him down, he never once surrendered to it. The two Bible scriptures that I think best define the way Trey handled his cancer are:

Have I not commanded you? Be strong and courageous. Do not be afraid; do not be discouraged, for the Lord your God will be with you wherever you go. (Joshua 1:9 NIV)

I can do all this through him who gives me strength. (Philippians 4:13 NIV)

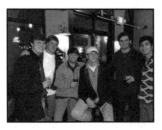

Trey and Sigma Chi brothers out in Athens, Georgia.

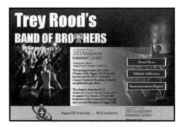

UGA Sigma Chi selected Dr. Hwu's melanoma research as their philanthropy for Derby Week Fundraiser.

August 2012 was Trey's two-year anniversary out from T-cell therapy. It was also his two-year anniversary in Sigma Chi, where he went on to serve on the pledge board as a trainer for the new fall class. At the first meeting, just as we had once been asked to do, he wanted the new guys to introduce themselves and share one interesting fact about their lives. To get the ball rolling, he told the guys he'd go first.

"I'm one of your pledge trainers," he told them. "My name is Trey Rood—and I defeated cancer."

I don't think anyone will ever forget that, either.

Wes

I was a junior at West Forsyth the year Trey started his freshman year at UGA. Even though he was busy with college, pledging, and trips to Houston, he came home for my Friday night football games. He did this both my junior and senior years, but was never happy to just hang out in the stands. He was usually down on the sidelines, watching all my plays, and scouting for Coach Rooney.

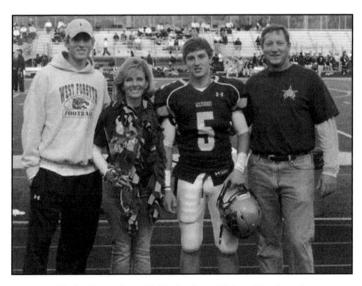

The family together with Wes for Senior Night at West Forsyth.

I graduated in the spring of 2012 and started classes that fall at the University of Mississippi in Oxford. Like so many of the men on dad's side of the family, I became a pledge of Sigma Chi, only I'm in the Eta chapter. In January 2013, Dad and Trey came to Oxford to attend the initiation ceremony. It was really great having them there.

Trey and I have always been close, but becoming Sigma Chi brothers gave us another thing to bond over. It has deepened what we already had, but there was still one thing that was even bigger and better. Trey's fight with melanoma brought me closer to Christ and I could see that it had done the same thing for Trey.

Through Him, we have our best brotherhood of all.

Chapter Eighteen

Cherie

For Charlie, Trey, Wes, and me, Christmas 2012 was so much merrier than the one just a year earlier. We had tried to celebrate that one amid so much uncertainty about Trey's health and whatever came next with the game plan. What a difference a year can make, though. Lights shone brighter, food tasted better, and carols sounded richer as we thanked God for Trey's latest report from MD Anderson. Hope encompassed the entire atmosphere in our home.

We were, however, very saddened by the passing of a young girl in our community who had fought a brave three-year battle with stage IV neuroblastoma cancer (a cancer affecting nerve tissue). Lily Anderson, who dreamed of becoming a country music singer (and sang the National Anthem before an Atlanta Braves game), was only eleven years old when she slipped away just before Christmas. Our community had supported many fundraisers for her just as they did for Trey, and she and Trey had become friends. I visited her shortly before her death. She had so many questions about Trey and how he had fought his cancer. I told her to never give up and was hoping Trey would get to visit her before Christmas. Sadly, we missed her funeral because we were in Houston.

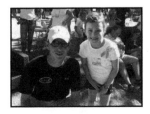

Trey connects with Lily Anderson, a young girl in the community who battled stage IV neuroblastoma cancer.

Shortly after the New Year, Trey and I, along with my sister Ann, had plans to visit MD Anderson on January 11 for a dedication ceremony of the Miriam and Jim Mulva Conference Center. In honor of their own son, who was an early-stage melanoma survivor, the Mulvas established a generous private fund to support melanoma research and other melanoma patients seeking care at MD Anderson. This proved to be a huge financial blessing to us, since Trey's trial was not being funded or supported by a pharmaceutical company. T-cell therapy is a scientific process of research to grow a patient's T-cells and develop the infusion process to put the cells back into the patient. It takes private funds to support this type of research, and the Mulvas were a big part of why Trey got his T-cells.

On January 10, though, my father passed away unexpectedly, a devastating and crushing loss to this lifelong daddy's girl. Initially, I considered cancelling our trip to Houston, but knowing how enthusiastic my father had been about us going, and we decided to travel as planned. It was very difficult for the three of us in light of our personal loss, but shortly after we arrived, I knew it had been the right decision.

That day, we learned that Trey is an MD Anderson rock star . . . and that this visit was about acknowledging that, as well as so much more. Dr. Hwu's office had scheduled a luncheon where we met the three brilliant lab technicians and supervising doctor who had overseen the growth of Trey's T-cells in the lab back in June 2010. We all seemed to be feeding off each other's excitement, going back and forth asking questions.

For us, it was fascinating listening to them describing the details and depth of literally growing Trey's T-cells. I felt such a connection with these people who worked hard to save Trey's life. They, on the other hand, had only known Trey as a cell. Now, here he was in the flesh—a tall, healthy, and

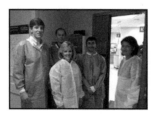

Trey and Cherie meet the doctor and lab technicians who oversaw Trey's T-cell growth.

happy young man. They wanted to hear all about what his life was like after the T-cell therapy.

We got to go on an amazing lab tour with all of them. It was incredible learning how many details had to fall exactly into place to assure that there would be a chance for the T-cells to grow. After putting on scrubs, plastic caps, and these roomy, white cover-ups that we called "moon suits," we got to see the bright, sterile facility where the cells are grown. We stepped through one chamber after another, each one becoming more sterile than the former, until we were standing among ten rooms that are used exclusively for cell growth.

Somewhere between these chambers was the room where Trey's cells had been protected, nurtured, and grown. When they showed us which one, we just couldn't believe it was a random coincidence that his cells had been grown in room number five—the same number as his treasured high school football jersey.

After the tour, we changed from our space-age medical outfits back into regular clothes and went to a meeting with Dr. Hwu. This time, we were in his administration office instead of the clinical office we had always seen him in. After a brief discussion with Dr. Hwu, taking a few pictures, and reliving some of Trey's treatments and medical experiences at MD Anderson, we headed to the 11th floor for the conference center dedication. Instead of the typical ribbon-cutting type of ceremony we were expecting, we were met with lights, cameras, and video at what appeared to be a press conference on the verge of starting. When Dr. Hwu approached us and said, "When I call you up . . . " we knew this was going to be more than we anticipated!

"We have to get up and talk?" Trey whispered to me. "Mom, what should I say?"

"Just speak from the heart," I answered, "and start with the day you first came here."

About twenty-five people were present. They included the Mulvas, the president of MD Anderson, Dr. Ronald DePinho, and other doctors and people from MD Anderson's business development department who were documenting what was about to be revealed as a celebration of Trey's life. We watched a PowerPoint presentation by Dr. Hwu that focused on the work he was doing with T-cell therapy. He called Trey an inspiration to "keep moving forward." Trey and I both spoke about how we had met Dr. Hwu and what he had given us. It was only about a five-minute talk between the two of us, and even got emotional at times, as we explained how all of them in that room had given Trey the "rest of his life." We talked about how we had come to MD Anderson, our connection to Dr. Hwu, the confidence and relationship we have with him, and why T-cell treatment was a life-changing experience for our family.

The official dedication of the conference center was followed by a full reception that included the lab technicians and the melanoma department. Everyone present swarmed around Trey, who was apparently a T-cell machine, having grown over one hundred billion of them when the norm is somewhere around fifty billion! As I watched him thank people and answer questions, I wondered if he—one of only ten patients at MD Anderson to receive dendritic cells during T-cell therapy—was a modern-day pioneer in the world of medical miracles. After all, every medical treatment that is now considered a standard cure or form of management was once in the same stages of research as Trey's trial.

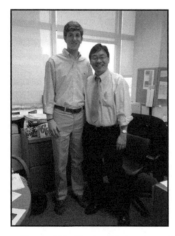 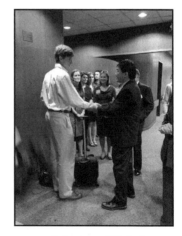

Trey and Dr. Hwu met before the conference center dedication at MD Anderson
(January 2013).

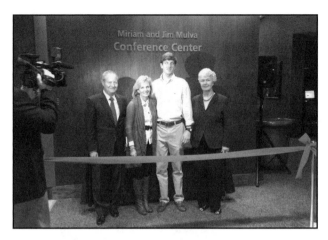

Trey and Cherie with the Mulva family, who made Trey's
T-cell treatment possible.

Is that why he was here? Is that why he had been through and done all the things he had done? Was this God's plan—the one Trey talks about? I honestly don't yet know the answers to those questions. Even if they were an absolute yes, would any parents wish for or choose this journey for their child? No, they wouldn't.

It was given to my child, though. He accepted it, but only because accepting its reality was the first step in fighting it. When Trey played football, he never downplayed the strength of an opponent. Instead, he focused on ways to win in spite of it. If one play didn't work, he would change the plan and re-enter the game with a new one.

When the opponent was the worst stage possible of melanoma, Trey never backed down, no matter how many times it came at him. He fought back with everything he had, which showed itself through grace, faith, and maturity that were well beyond his years and scope of life experience. So while I never wanted this path for Trey, I can see why he was chosen to show others how to walk it. He plays to win. One of his football coaches said, "God doesn't choose the qualified; He qualifies the chosen." We have a "Pray for Trey" plaque with this very saying on it that hangs in our home.

Our family hopes to send a message of positivity, because the people who are positive are most likely to keep seeking answers and options that lead to the next win. If the opponent is playing hard, and your defense strategies aren't working, change the game plan—as many times as you need to.

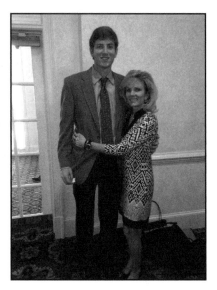

*Trey and Cherie together at a Sigma Chi
Mother's Luncheon.*

Trey

On any field of life, melanoma was the toughest opponent I ever faced. Today, I believe that it's behind me. Every return to MD Anderson serves only as confirmation that cancer is no longer in the game.

Family, friends, coaches, teachers, youth leaders, people in the community—there are so many people I am thankful for. I'm grateful to Dr. Hwu for wanting to bring hope to those who hear the word "melanoma." I'm grateful for parents who wouldn't give up or leave any stone unturned. I'm glad to have a brother man enough to understand my needs.

Mostly, I'm grateful for God, who put all the right people in place so that I could get well. He's the reason I'm still here, but He sure gave me a great team He could work through. At some point, He showed me that this story wasn't just about me. I'm not sure when I realized it, but I know that this journey became an opportunity as well as a fight. It was an opportunity to inspire others and play a part in taking this disease down.

There was nothing random about ending up at MD Anderson. It was all part of a strategic plan. Even though it had its tests of faith, it also had its rewards for standing firm. I think that being an inspiration to others and a pioneer patient in a new melanoma treatment were my callings in all of this, what I needed to live out.

We had to change the game plan several times during the years I was at war with melanoma. I guess it's like that with a lot of things in life. Everything needs a plan, but if it doesn't work the first time, some people throw in the towel, thinking it must not be "meant to be." Others search for a different way, and sometimes even find choices they didn't know were there until they looked. Sometimes the first game plan is the only one you need. If it's not, don't be afraid to change it. In other words, never give up.

Remember, God is always obviously organized for those who can trust, believe, and never give up hope. The God-things in my life were, and are, a great illustration of this.

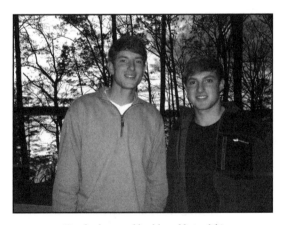

Trey back to good health and living life!

Afterword
by Dr. Patrick Hwu

It is a true honor for myself and my team at MD Anderson to have been involved in the care of this special young man and his remarkable family. Trey was indeed facing a daunting opponent, and the courage he displayed in going through his challenging therapies has been inspirational. Melanoma, a cancer that starts in the body's pigment cells of the skin, can attack people of all ages. Of all the types of skin cancers, melanoma is the deadliest, because it can readily spread to all parts of the body. Once it spreads, it is very hard to cure. However, steady progress is being made, and a number of clinical trials are starting to show success in treating these advanced cases in some patients.

One of these new therapies is T-cell therapy. In most melanoma tumors, the immune system is "trying to work" in that T-cells, capable of directly killing cancer cells, are present in the tumor. However, the tumors continue to grow, either because not enough T-cells are present or because they are being suppressed by the cancer (cancers can make a number of substances that can act like "kryptonite" against the defending T-cells). We have learned to take tumors to the laboratory and grow out the T-cells to billions in number, then give them back to the patients to try to get their tumors to shrink. Each patient gets back their own cells, because only their cells can recognize and kill their particular tumors. Although we have had good results in some patients, we are still trying to improve this therapy.

A few years ago, one of our trainees, Dr. Yanyan Lou, found in mouse models that giving the T-cells, followed by stimulation of the T-cells with a dendritic cell vaccine, could improve the results compared to the T-cells alone. With support from the National Cancer Institute, as well as donors such as Jim and Miriam Mulva, we took this concept from the laboratory to the clinic. Trey was one of our first patients to get both the T-cells and the dendritic cells. Despite the success in our mouse models, we never know how any of our new therapies will be tolerated in patients, or how effective they will be. Therefore, it was with considerable courage that Trey embarked on this "change in the game plan." We shared with Trey and his family that we didn't know how well this combination of T-cells and dendritic cells would be tolerated in people. Besides treatment side effects, it was also exhausting for Trey and his family to make the arduous trips back and forth to Houston. I can truly say that I have always been impressed by their stamina, determination, and love for one another. I know having the backing of so many who loved him, his family, football team, school, and the many who wore the "Pray for Trey" wristbands, had a lot to do with Trey's winning scrimmages against melanoma. I conclude that this was likely the toughest season any young athlete could have faced, and he faced it well.

Trey received 107 billion T-cells and two doses of 167 million dendritic cells. Growing this number of cells in the laboratory is very labor-intensive and we are very fortunate to have dedicated, highly trained personnel that are committed and willing to work long hours to generate these therapies for patients. This includes Dr. Laszlo Radvanyi, Dr. Chantale Bernatchez, Orenthial Fulbright, Rahmatu Mansaray, Chris Toth, Renjith Ramachandran, Seth Wardell, and Audrey Gonzalez.

We are very pleased at the wonderful response we are seeing in Trey, as well as in other patients on our trials. Our next steps are two-fold. We would like to improve the therapy further, and are working to put genes into the T-cells so they can more efficiently migrate into the tumor, and we are also working on other genes to make the cells more resistant to the "kryptonite" made by the tumors. Importantly, we are working toward simplifying the growth process to allow this therapy to be administered at many other centers in the world. Currently, only a few other centers, such as the National Cancer Institute in Bethesda, Maryland, offer this type of therapy.

In addition, there are other new treatments on the horizon for melanoma that are giving us further hope. Ipilimumab, an antibody that takes the "brakes" off of immune cells, is a drug that was recently approved by the United States Food and Drug Administration (FDA) for the treatment of advanced melanoma. We were trying to give this drug to Trey, but at the time, it was only available as part of a clinical trial that would not allow participation by patients with brain metastases. This is a tough situation that we often face in the clinic, and in my opinion, we need to find better ways to get new therapies to patients more quickly. It took over ten years to get ipilimumab FDA-approved, and this is just too long. If a drug appears effective, even in a subset of patients, and the disease has a dire prognosis, why not approve it sooner? There are now even more effective drugs in this class (such as anti-PD1), and it is my hope that their approval comes quickly for all the patients that need it, but may not meet the criteria or cannot find an open clinical trial.

The other major recent advance in the treatment of advanced melanoma is the development of targeted therapies. These are small molecular drugs that can turn off the mutations or "light switches" that activate the tumor's "circuitry." For patients with a mutation in the gene *BRAF*, for example, there is now an FDA-approved pill that works in most patients to shrink their tumors. Unfortunately, it only works for a few months in most patients. Future goals are to use these pills in combination with other pills targeting additional "light switches," or in combination with immune therapies, such as T-cells or the antibodies discussed previously. In the end, the best therapies will likely consist of combinations of targeted and immunotherapies. Trey's tumor, however, did not have the *BRAF* mutation. Instead, it had a mutation in a gene called *NRAS*. Today, we don't have effective targeted therapies for *NRAS*-positive tumors, but there are hints from mouse models that may lead us toward effective therapies for this kind of tumor, and we are planning to start new clinical trials are in progress that are testing these concepts.

Trey's story provides the opportunity to increase the awareness of melanoma and to educate regarding the most effective prevention methods. We still don't understand how melanoma starts in all cases, and are not able to prevent all of them. However, we do know that ultraviolet rays from the sun, and in particular, sun burns, can increase the chances of getting melanoma. For this reason, we encourage people to stay out of the sun during the hottest parts of the day, to use sunscreen and protective clothing, and to avoid sun burns. In addition, because melanoma is sometimes curable when caught early, we encourage people to see a dermatologist on a regular basis, especially if a mole seems to be changing.

Trey's story is one of courage, love, and inspiration. It also highlights the importance of cancer research to society. There has been tremendous progress in the last decade in the science and understanding of our immune system and cancer. We are well poised to make very significant strides in the near future, but this can only be accomplished if we as a society work together to provide the adequate focus and funding. Trey's story illustrates that research breakthroughs can have a very high impact on patients and their families. It further shows that the love of family and friends is essential during times of crisis. Although we are doing better today in patients with advanced melanoma like Trey's, we still only cure a fraction of patients. With continued research, we hope that one day soon all patients with cancer will respond as well as Trey has.

———

Follow Trey's continuing melanoma survival journey: www.prayfortrey.org.